LEARNING ABOUT LUPUS:

A USER FRIENDLY GUIDE

Second Edition

Editor
Mary E. Moore, PhD, MD

Associate Editors
Peter E. Callegari, MD
Jay A. Denbo, DDS
Carolyn McGrory, MS, RN

44 West Lancaster Avenue
Ardmore, PA 19003
(610) 649-9202

Library of Congress Catalog Card Number: 97-73837
Published by
MainLine DeskTop Publishing Company
5 Great Valley Parkway, Suite 274
Malvern, PA 19355
Printed in the U.S.A.
ISBN 0-9659530-0-9

ACKNOWLEDGMENTS

The Board of Directors of the Lupus Foundation of Delaware Valley wishes to express its deep appreciation to the members of their Medical Advisory Board who made the publication of this book possible. We are also grateful to editors, Mary E. Moore, PhD, MD; Peter Callegari, MD; Jay A. Denbo, DDS and Carolyn McGrory, MS, RN, for the long hours they spent in the editing process. Special thanks are due to Mary E. Moore, PhD, MD for providing the drive and dedication necessary to see a project of this complexity to its conclusion. We also thank Anne Bagshaw, MSc for her conscientious supervision of the entire production process.

DEDICATION

Publication of this book is made possible by a bequest from the estate of Betty Rothstein, and is dedicated to the memory of her beloved daughter, Ruthie.

CONTRIBUTING AUTHORS:

Mary P. Brassell, MA, CRRN
Rehabilitation Manager
BAYADA Nurses
Moorestown, NJ

Peter Callegari, MD
Assistant Professor of Medicine
Chief, Clinical Services
Division of Rheumatology
Hospital of the University of PA
Philadelphia, PA

Edmund T. Carroll, DO
Professor of Medicine
Allergy & Immunology
Philadelphia College of
    Osteopathic Medicine
Philadelphia, PA

Douglas B. Cines, MD
Professor of Pathology
Laboratory Medicine & Medicine
Hospital of the University of PA
Philadelphia, PA

Ernesto L. Collazo, MD
Senior Clinical Instructor
Department of Ophthalmology
Hahnemann University
Philadelphia, PA

Raphael J. DeHoratius, MD
Professor of Medicine
Director, Lupus Study Center
Thomas Jefferson University
Philadelphia, PA

Jay A. Denbo, DDS
Associate Professor of
    Periodontology
Temple University School of
    Dentistry
Philadelphia, PA

Bertram Greenspun, DO
Clinical Associate Professor
Department of Rehabilitation
    Medicine
Thomas Jefferson University
    Hospital
Philadelphia, PA

Bruce I. Hoffman, MD
Associate Professor of Medicine
Chief, Division of Rheumatology
Medical College of Pennsvlvania
Philadelphia, PA

Sandra Koffler, PhD
Associate Professor
Departments of Psychiatry &
    Neurology
Allegheny University Hospitals
Hahnemann Division
Philadelphia, PA

Michael M. Margolin, M.D.
Neurological Center
Willingboro, NJ

Carolyn H. McGrory, MS, RN
Research Coordinator
Rheumatology/Transplant Surgery
Thomas Jefferson University
    Hospital
Philadelphia, PA

Mary E. Moore, PhD, MD
Attending in Rheumatology
Albert Einstein Medical Center
Professor of Medicine
Temple University School of
  Medicine
Philadelphia, PA

Barbara E. Ostrov, MD
Associate Professor of Pediatrics
  & Medicine
Pediatric & Adult Rheumatology
Penn State University School
  of Medicine
Milton S. Hershey Medical Center
Hershey, PA

Louis J. Riley, Jr., MD
Professor & Chairman
Department of Medicine
Morehouse School of Medicine
Atlanta, GA

Stephen H. Sinclair, M.D.
Clinical Professor of
  Ophthalmology
Allegheny University of the Health
  Sciences
Hahnemann Division
Philadelphia, PA

Phyllis Slutsky, RN, MEd
Pediatric Rheumatology Nurse
  Specialist
Children's Hospital of Philadelphia
Dept. of Homecare
Philadelphia, PA

Sheldon Solomon, MD
Arthritis & Rheumatic Disease
  Associates
Cherry Hill, NJ

Marvin E. Steinberg, MD
Professor & Vice Chairman
Department of Orthopaedic Surgery
Director, Joint Reconstruction Center
Hospital of the University of PA
Philadelphia, PA

James L. Stinnett, MD
Professor of Psychiatry
Hospital of the University of PA
Philadelphia, PA

Alan G. Wasserstein, MD
Associate Professor of Medicine
Renal Electrolyte & Hypertension
  Division
Hospital of the University of PA
Philadelphia, PA

Guy F. Webster, MD, PhD
Associate Professor
Departments of Dermatology &
  Internal Medicine
Thomas Jefferson University
  Hospital
Philadelphia, PA

Ronald Wapner, MD
Director, Maternal Fetal Medicine
Thomas Jefferson University
Philadelphia, PA

Burton Zweiman, MD
Chief, Allergy & Immunology
Professor of Medicine
Hospital of the University of PA
Philadelphia, PA

PREFACE TO THE SECOND EDITION

In 1991, the lupus Foundation of Delaware Valley produced the first edition of *Learning About Lupus: A User Friendly Guide*. Judging from the number of copies sold and the enthusiastic response of readers, we concluded that our efforts had been successful. Six years later, however, knowledge about lupus has increased and new methods of treatment are now available. We therefore decided that it was time to publish a second edition of our book.

Coincidentally, just when we were thinking about a new edition (and wondering how to keep the price very low but at the same time improve the quality of the production), we were the beneficiaries of some good fortune. We received an unrestricted bequest from the estate of Betty Rothstein. Mrs. Rothstein wanted to honor the memory of her beloved daughter, who had died of lupus, at a very young age. Because our Board of Directors felt there was no better way to use this money than to increase public awareness of lupus and promote education concerning the disease, it determined to use this bequest to subsidize this second edition.

Once we decided to update *Learning About Lupus: A User Friendly Guide*, our Medical Advisory Board, whose members had written the first edition, responded with enthusiasm. They determined that not only would they update information, but that they would attempt to improve the contents in other ways. What they produced is a book which is improved over the first edition. They have included more tables and figures, highlighted key points in special text boxes, expanded existing chapters, and have added two new chapters: Chapter Two explores in some detail aspects of lupus not featured in chapters of their own, including muscle, heart and gastrointestinal disease. Chapter Twenty One, the other new chapter, repeats questions commonly asked by patients and other concerned laypeople, answering them in understandable, nontechnical language.

As I stated in the Preface to the First Edition, my own struggle with lupus has been a long and very difficult one. I continue to believe that one of the most important factors in my continuing effort to survive lupus and its complications has been the result of my efforts at self-education. When I was first diagnosed two decades ago, there was very little written on lupus for the layperson. Today the situation is vastly improved; there are currently many books, pamphlets, videos and newsletters available. We encourage lupus patients to learn as much as they can about their disease. We think our book offers a valuable addition to the literature that will allow them to do just this.

Ruth M. Zeit
President, Lupus Foundation of Delaware Valley, Inc.
Ardmore, Pennsylvania

CONTENTS

CHAPTER 1. AN INTRODUCTION

Mary E. Moore, PhD, MD and
Edmund T. Carroll, DO

Systemic lupus erythematosus (SLE or lupus) is a disease which can affect many parts of the body and cause many different symptoms. Among adults, lupus is nine times more common in females than males. Lupus most commonly affects people between the ages of twenty to forty and thus occurs most frequently in women during their child-bearing years. An African American woman is three times more likely than a Caucasian woman to be affected. Children and teenagers can also get lupus. During the first ten years of life, girls will get lupus three to seven times more often than boys. (Childhood lupus is the subject of Chapter 15.)

African American women are 3 times more likely than Caucasian women to get lupus.

The cause of lupus is not known. The immune system, nature's means of protecting the body from foreign invaders such as viruses and bacteria, overreacts in lupus. Normally when an invader enters the body, the immune system responds by turning on the action of white blood cells called lymphocytes. Some of these cells, known as B lym-

Sunlight, hormones and certain medicines can "trigger" SLE in some people.

1

phocytes, begin to produce antibodies which can serve as weapons against the invader. Other lymphocytes, known as T lymphocytes, help to control the action of the B lymphocytes. In lupus, for reasons we do yet fully understand, T lymphocytes don't perform properly and B lymphocytes are activated inappropriately. As a result, antibodies are produced against a great

---

Table I. ACR CRITERIA FOR THE CLASSIFICATION OF LUPUS*

1. Malar rash (red rash over the cheeks and nose)
2. Discoid lupus (distinctive patchy, scaling, skin rash)
3. Photosensitivity (rash or illness after sun exposure)
4. Oral or nasal ulcers (shallow sores in the nose and mouth)
5. Arthritis (pain and swelling in the joints)
6. Serositis (inflammation causing pain involving the coverings of the lung or heart, or the lining of the abdomen)
7. Certain types of kidney problems which may cause blood or protein in the urine
8. Neurologic problems showing up as seizures or mental illness
9. Hematologic disorders (low counts of various types of blood cells)
10. Immunologic disorders manifested by abnormal blood tests:
    (a) positive L.E. test; (b) anti-DNA antibody; (c) anti-Smith antibody; (d) false positive test for syphilis (See Chapter 3)
11. A positive antinuclear antibody (see Chapter 3)

* It is suggested that a person may be classified as having lupus if he or she has four or more of the eleven criteria.

---

number of substances including some of the body's own tissues. These antibodies which are destructive to the body itself are known as "autoantibodies".

What triggers the immune system in lupus to over-react has not been discovered. We do know that people can inherit a tendency to react in this way to certain things in the environment. (The inherited or genetic aspects of SLE are the subject of Chapter 4). The things which set off SLE in genetically vulnerable people are sometimes called "triggers". For years a search has gone on to find a virus which might act as a trigger for lupus. Although many experts feel strongly that one or more viruses may act to trigger SLE, no such virus has been identified so far. What is clear, however, is that other things in the environment can trigger lupus. These include sunlight, hormones, and certain medications.

To aid in the diagnosis of lupus, the American College of Rheumatology (ACR) has listed various criteria shown in Table 1 to guide the physician in identifying lupus. These guidelines are based on the patient's complaints, the doctor's findings when examining the patient, and the patient's laboratory test results. The criteria include the things that are most typical of lupus as compared to other similar diseases. They do not include all, or even the most common, problems a patient with lupus may experience. For example, people with lupus very frequently suffer from fatigue, fevers, muscle and joint aching, swollen glands, and generalized feelings of being unwell. None of these complaints are listed as part of the criteria, however, because they occur in many other diseases besides SLE. It is also true that not all patients with SLE will have all of the problems listed in the

No two patients with lupus will have an illness which is exactly alike.

criteria. Each person with lupus tends to have his or her own disease pattern. This is often established early in the disease and may continue for many years. For example, one lupus patient may have only skin problems, anemia and fever. Another may have only arthritis, pleuritis (inflammation of the covering of the lung and the chest cavity) and a decline in the small blood cells called platelets. In fact, no two patients with lupus will have exactly the same disease. For this reason, people with lupus should avoid attempting to predict the course of their own disease by comparing themselves to others with SLE.

The first criterion for lupus involves the skin. The best known skin problem in lupus is the "butterfly" rash. This is a red rash over the cheeks and the bridge of the nose (the malar area). Not all skin changes in this area are due to lupus. Many people experience a normal flushing of the cheeks; sunburn typically affects this area and some skin diseases such as acne rosacea are found over the cheeks and the bridge of the nose.

Other skin problems listed among the lupus criteria are a "discoid" rash (slightly raised patches of skin which have a definite reddish border, are associated with scaling, and develop a paler-than-normal color in their center), sun sensitivity (rash after exposure to sunlight), and oral ulcers (small raw areas where the normal lining of the mouth is absent). In addition, many other skin problems are common in lupus. These include alopecia (hair loss), many different kinds of rashes, changes in the tiny blood vessels (capillaries) around the finger nails, and a widespread purple network pattern of blood vessels (livedo reticularis) often prominent over the legs. (See Chapter 6 for more about the skin in lupus.)

The fifth lupus criterion deals with arthritis. Almost all lupus patients have joint pains at some time during their illness, and many have arthritis or joint inflammation (swelling, warmth, redness, or tenderness). The type of arthritis associated with lupus is similar to that seen in rheumatoid arthritis but it is not usually as severe, does not cause a wearing away of the bone, and does not result in deformity. Lupus arthritis most commonly affects the hands, the wrists, the knees, and the feet. Sometimes patients with lupus, especially those on corticosteroids, have involvement of the bone due to a loss of blood supply. This is called "avascular necrosis". When this occurs in the bone near a joint (most commonly the hip), damage to the joint may result in what is called degenerative or osteoarthritis. (Chapter 13 discusses more about bone involvement in lupus.)

Serositis, the sixth item on the list of criteria, is a general term for inflammation of the delicate tissues which cover certain internal organs and line the body compartments. It is quite common in lupus. When serositis affects a particular organ, it is given a specific name. For example, inflammation of the tissue (the pleura) which lines the chest cavity and covers the lungs is called pleuritis. Inflammation of the covering of the heart (the pericardium) is called pericarditis. Movement of the tissues affected by serositis, for example, taking a deep breath when pleuritis is present, may cause pain. The doctor can often hear a characteristic scraping sound called a "rub", when listening over the involved areas with a stethoscope. Abdominal pain in lupus is sometimes caused by inflammation of the covering of the intestines and the lining of the abdominal cavity (peritonitis). This kind of pain can be very severe and can imitate diverticulitis, appendicitis, etc. Fluid sometimes accumulates in a body cavity as a result of serositis. If it causes pain or interferes with function, it may have to be withdrawn.

One of the most complicated problems in lupus, and also one of the criteria, is kidney disease. Kidney involvement can be detected in about 50% of SLE patients. It varies from very mild involvement, which causes the patient no symptoms, to severe disease requiring special treatment. Doctors detect early kidney problems by finding protein or red blood cells in the patient's urine. They may ask the patient to collect 24-hour urine samples. These help the doctor to make more accurate estimates of how well the kidney is working. At times it may be necessary to obtain a biopsy (a tiny piece of kidney tissue) to discover the type and extent of damage which is present. (Lupus, as it involves the kidney, is further discussed in Chapter 7).

The central nervous system may be involved by

SLE. Such involvement may cause a variety of disorders. These can range from a mild feeling of nervousness, to problems with concentration and memory loss, to seizures and involuntary movements, and rarely to mental illness or stroke. Only the more serious of these meet the criterion for central nervous system lupus. Since very similar nervous problems can result from some medications, infection, hardening of the arteries, or unrelated mental illness, and since there is no one test for central nervous system lupus, the central nervous system lupus criterion is often difficult to apply. (Neurologic problems seen in lupus are discussed in more detail in Chapter 8. Neuropsychological testing is discussed in Chapter 9 and psychological problems associated with lupus are discussed in Chapter 10.)

The last three of the ACR criteria involve abnormal blood test results. One of the frequent disorders in lupus is a decrease in the number of white blood cells, especially the lymphocytes. Since some of the drugs used to treat lupus can cause a decrease in the white blood cell count, monitoring the safe use of these drugs may, at times, be complicated. The platelet is another blood cell frequently decreased in lupus. Platelets play a key role in blood clotting, and having too few platelets can lead to problems with bleeding. Anemia, a decrease in the number of red blood cells, is almost always present to some extent in cases of active lupus. Anemia may result from a failure of a lupus patient's bone marrow to manufacture red blood cells, or from bleeding caused by a low platelet count, or from the destruction of red blood cells by antibodies. (More about the changes of the blood cells in lupus in Chapter 12.)

In SLE, the B lymphocytes are stimulated to manufacture many different antibodies including so-called "autoantibodies".

Lupus may overlap rheumatoid arthritis, scleroderma, or dermatomyositis.

These target the patient's own tissues. The body, in essence, attacks itself! In addition to the widely known antinuclear antibody (ANA), there are many other autoantibodies which may be present and which may aid in the diagnosis of lupus. (See Chapter 3 on the role of laboratory tests in lupus diagnosis).

Lupus may be difficult at times to distinguish from other connective tissue diseases causing problems in classification. Rheumatoid arthritis typically involves a similar, though usually more severe, arthritis with morning stiffness. Patients with rheumatoid arthritis may have a positive ANA in addition to a positive test for an antibody known as the rheumatoid factor. Scleroderma (also called systemic sclerosis) usually is associated with Raynaud's phenomenon (see Chapter 2), arthritis and a positive ANA but is characterized by the development of firm, tight skin. Dermatomyositis involves a facial rash and may be associated with arthritis and lung disease, but marked muscle weakness is the main feature. Overlapping features of lupus and rheumatoid arthritis, dermatomyositis, or scleroderma are not uncommon. When features overlap, some cases are referred to as undifferentiated connective tissue disease or mixed connective tissue disease. Patients with overlap disease often get confused because different names for their diagnoses may be used by different doctors. Fortunately, treatment of these overlap cases is based on what features are present and what laboratory tests are abnormal and does not depend upon the name the disease is given. Since there is currently no cure for any of these diseases, the important thing is not how the disease manifestations are classified but whether they are treated appropriately.

Pregnancy is an occasion for special concern to the patient with SLE. It is very important for a woman with lupus who is planning a pregnancy to consult with her physician concerning her intentions. While pregnancy does not appear to affect the overall life expectancy of the lupus patient, lupus may flare during pregnancy. There is also an increase in premature births and stillbirths among lupus patients. Certain autoantibodies and other factors may be present in the blood of some women with lupus and are associated with these problems. If she finds herself with an unplanned pregnancy, a woman with lupus should seek medical help as soon as possible with an obstetrician experienced in dealing with high-risk cases. (This topic is covered in Chapter 18.)

Certain commonly used drugs may cause the body to make antinuclear antibodies and also may cause a mild form of lupus known as drug-induced lupus. Drug-induced lupus is characterized by **Some drugs cause a mild form of lupus.** joint pain and arthritis, fever, and pleuritis. Kidney and central nervous system involvement typically do not occur. Drugs which have been commonly associated with drug-induced lupus include: hydralazine and methyldopa (used to treat high blood pressure); isoniazid (used to treat tuberculosis); procainamide and quinidine (used to treat irregular heartbeat and, in the case of the latter, muscle cramps); and chlorpromazine (used to treat severe mental illness) severe hiccups, and persistent nausea and vomiting. Because of the possible effects of these drugs, it is important to know what medications a patient diagnosed as having lupus has been taking.

The treatment of SLE is variable. Some patients with lupus require very little treatment. Patients with drug-induced lupus may only need to have the offending drug stopped. Other lupus patients may need only steroid skin creams or ointments and sunscreens. Still others may require the use of simple pain medications and mild anti-inflammatory medicines such as aspirin and other nonsteroidal anti-inflammatory drugs (NSAIDS) for muscle pain or arthritis. Drugs such as hydroxychloroquine (a drug first used to treat malaria) are often used for lupus involving arthritis and skin disease. Adrenal corticosteroid drugs (steroids) given by mouth or intravenously are usually reserved for the more serious cases of SLE involving kidney or central nervous system disorders, certain blood cell problems, or serositis. To supplement steroids or to replace them when they don't work, immunosuppressive drugs, originally developed for use in cancer treatment ("chemotherapy"), have also been found to be helpful in treating lupus. (These and other medical treatments are described further in Chapter 5.)

In addition to medical treatment, there are other important considerations in the treatment of lupus. A well-balanced diet is essential to maximize health. There is no special diet which has proven to be useful for

Survival in lupus has increased greatly over recent years.

treating lupus, however. Clubs and support groups are available to offer education and psychological help. (See Chapter 19.) Physical and occupational therapy and other methods used in rehabilitation medicine can provide pain relief and can help to maintain function (discussed in Chapter 16). Psychotherapy and counseling can be an important addition to other forms of treatment and are available from different sources including psychiatrists, psychologists, and social workers. (These are discussed in Chapter 10 and mentioned in association with sexual dysfunction in Chapter 17.) Finally, one of the most helpful aspects of a treatment program is a good doctor-patient relationship. This will be the subject of an entire chapter later on (Chapter 20).

Over the years, we have had more and more success in the treatment of lupus. Studies done at Johns Hopkins University back in 1954 showed a survival rate in SLE less than 50% after four years. Several large studies done in the 1980's, however, revealed that 87% of lupus patients survived at least 5 years and 78% were still surviving after 10 years. A study of 570 lupus patients reported from New York City in 1991 described even further improvement with 93% (more than 9 out of 10!) of the group alive after 10 years. There is good reason to believe that this upward trend will continue as we learn more about lupus and how to control it.

CHAPTER 2. MORE ABOUT LUPUS

Bruce I. Hoffman, MD

In Chapter 1, we presented an introduction to SLE. Later in this book we will devote separate chapters to several of the major organ systems involved in lupus. These include the skin, the nervous system, the kidney, and the reproductive system. In the present chapter we will discuss problems which the patient with lupus may encounter in several other areas. Specifically, we will talk about the joints and the muscles, the heart and the circulation of the blood, the lungs, the gastrointestinal tract, and the immune system. In addition to addressing problems caused by the disease itself, we will mention some of the common problems in these areas caused by medications used to treat SLE.

The Joints

Involvement of the joints is the most common feature of lupus and is often the first sign of lupus which comes to the patient's attention. Joint problems in lupus usually take the form of ar-

The arthritis of lupus is usually mild.

thritis (from the Greek, meaning inflammation of the joint). Lupus arthritis usually causes pain when the joint is moved and the affected joint may become warm and swollen. Often, the knuckles of the fingers are affected but many other joints may be involved as well. The arthritis usually includes both the right and left sides of the body similarly and causes more discomfort first thing in the morning. The symptoms of lupus arthritis resemble those of rheumatoid arthritis but are usually much milder. Lupus arthritis does not destroy bone and is not crippling in the way that rheumatoid arthritis sometimes is. Early in the course of disease, it may be difficult to tell lupus arthritis and rheumatoid arthritis apart. At times a period of observation is necessary before the diagnosis can be made with certainty.

The arthritis in lupus is most often easy to control with nonsteroidal anti-inflammatory drugs, antimalarial drugs, or low dose steroids. If one joint is particularly troublesome, steroids are sometimes injected directly into the joint. Methotrexate, commonly used in rheumatoid arthritis, has been used to control the more severe cases of lupus arthritis.

At times, the fingers in a patient with lupus become somewhat crooked but are not painful. Although the fingers cannot be actively straightened out under their own power, they are easily straightened temporarily using another hand, a fact which the doctor often checks during the examination. These finger deformities do not represent arthritis. The problem is called "Jaccoud's arthropathy", named after a man who first noticed a similar problem in patients with rheumatic fever. It occurs because the supporting tissues of the joints become stretched. No medical treatment is needed. Hand function in Jaccoud's arthropathy is usually maintained but sometimes surgery is necessary to correct the deformities.

The Muscles

Aching of the muscles occurs very commonly in lupus. It often increases when the disease flares but is not itself a sign of any serious problem. Muscle aching can usually be relieved by the use of nonsteroidal anti-inflammatory medication.

Inflammation of the muscles, myositis, occurs rarely in lupus. When it is present, the patient's main complaint is one of weakness, most severe in the shoulders and the thighs. It may be difficult to work with raised arms, to carry heavy objects, to climb stairs, and to arise from a low seat. The muscle inflammation is confirmed by finding an

Weak muscles may indicate lupus activity or the effects of steroids.

elevation in a blood test called the creatine kinase (CK), by noting abnormalities on an electromyogram (EMG), and by finding certain changes on a small sample of muscle obtained at a biopsy. Myositis is usually well treated with corticosteroids which reduce the inflammation. Treatment is monitored by following the CK blood levels which will fall as muscle strength gradually returns to normal. A maintenance dose of steroid is sometimes required to maintain control of the inflammation.

Muscle weakness is also a common side effect of steroid use. This is called "steroid myopathy". The severity of the weakness, and the amount of medication that causes it, varies from one person to another. Steroid myopathy is usually most noticeable in the upper leg muscles. The CK blood test is normal in steroid myopathy and the diagnosis is often made simply by observing improvement in strength when the steroid dose is reduced. Even when the weakness is severe, normal muscle function can be restored.

The Heart And Circulation

The heart can be affected in several ways by SLE. Lupus can cause inflammation of the covering around the heart, damage to the heart muscle or to the heart valves (the delicate flaps in the heart that help direct the flow of blood).

Pericarditis

The sac which covers the heart is called the pericardium and inflammation of this sac is called pericarditis. Pericarditis is very common in people with lupus. It leads to pain in the chest which may come and go. The pain is often mild but can be severe and cause concern about a heart attack. Pericarditis pain is sharp and is located behind the breast bone. It is relieved by sitting up and leaning forward. (In contrast, the pain of a heart attack is typically like a very strong pressure, is not relieved by any special position, and is often accompanied by sweating and a feeling of being sick to one's stomach.)

Pericarditis is diagnosed in several ways. When the doctor listens to the heart a rubbing sound can sometimes be heard. Two tests which aid in diagnosis are the electrocardiogram which records the electrical activity of the heart and the echocardiogram which makes a picture with sound waves of the heart muscle and valve motion. The echocardiogram can show if fluid is present in the heart sac. This is usually a small amount and poses no danger. On those rare occasions when a large amount of fluid is detected, it may have to be drained and an operation performed to prevent it from forming again. Pericarditis is usually easy to treat with nonsteroidal anti-inflammatory medicines or prednisone.

Myocarditis and Endocarditis

Much less common than pericarditis is inflammation of the heart muscle itself, myocarditis. In the case of myocarditis the heart function may decline and the patients may note difficulty breathing while exerting themselves and while lying flat in bed. They may awaken at night due to difficulty breathing and experience irregular heart beats and swelling of the ankles due to retention of body fluid. Myocarditis is diagnosed by the finding of an elevated amount of a certain type of CK enzyme (in this case, the special type which comes from heart muscle), and by abnormal electrocardiograms and echocardiograms. Myocarditis is treated with corticosteroids and typically requires evaluation and treatment by a cardiologist.

It has recently been recognized that lupus can also affect the valves of the heart (endocarditis) more commonly than had been thought to be the case. Valvular disease may cause a sound known as a heart murmur which the doctor can hear with a stethoscope and is accurately detected by an echocardiogram. It is very rare for lupus valve disease to result in poor heart function but the heart valves can become scarred. The scarred valves are more apt than healthy valves to become infected by germs which get into the blood stream. People known to have scarred valves are advised to take antibiotics when undergoing certain dental and surgical procedures which may cause germs to be introduced into the blood circulation.

Cholesterol and Heart Attacks

Cholesterol is a normal component of the fat that circulates in the blood but an elevated cholesterol level is an important risk factor for coronary artery disease (blockage of the arteries supplying blood to the heart) leading to heart attacks. Doctors have known for some time that people with longstanding lupus have

People with lupus have an increased risk of heart disease.

an increased risk of heart attacks. Some studies have shown that a person with lupus is nine times as likely as a healthy person to suffer a heart attack. This increased risk is due to the effects of the disease itself as well as to the complications of treatment.

The ideal cholesterol reading is below 200. Moreover, a large portion of the cholesterol should be a type known as high density lipoprotein (HDL). The HDL is believed to have a protective effect on the development of fat deposits in the blood vessels and is sometimes referred to by the layman as the "good cholesterol". When the cholesterol level is checked, it is possible for the doctor to determine the amount of HDL present and also the amount of low density lipoprotein (LDL), the cholesterol component that correlates with coronary artery disease.

In the case of otherwise healthy persons, the usual cause of dangerous levels of cholesterol in the blood is too much fat in the diet or a tendency, inherited from their parents, to deal with fat in their bodies in an abnormal manner. In the case of lupus, there are additional factors at work. Lupus itself may cause kidney disease and lupus is often treated with corticosteroids, both of which factors can raise the levels of dangerous fats in the blood. Lupus patients also often have high blood pressure and abnormal proteins in the blood which can increase the damage that fat can do to the arteries. It is therefore very important that elevated cholesterol levels in lupus patients be detected and treated in order to lower risk for heart attack.

A diet low in fat is the first step in treatment. A session with a dietitian is often helpful in achieving this. Weight loss and exercise also play a role in treatment. If these kinds of changes alone are ineffective in lowering abnormal fat levels, it is necessary to add medications. These drugs actually change the way the body handles fats.

Raynaud's Phenomenon

SLE can also affect small arteries. One of the most commonly recognized of these effects is Raynaud's phenomenon. Raynaud's phenomenon is caused by a spasm of the arteries, the vessels which bring oxygen-rich blood to the body. Patients usually complain of Raynaud's in the fingers but it can occur in the toes and occasionally in the ears, nose, and even in internal organs. The spasm typically happens in response to cold but can also occur in response to stress (when someone is upset or nervous). When a finger is affected by Raynaud's, it first turns white as the blood drains out of it. Later, when the tissue in the finger becomes starved for oxygen, the finger turns bluish in color. The affected finger also becomes painful. As the circulation is restored, usually through warming, the finger often turns red.

Not everyone with Raynaud's has, or will ever get, SLE. Some have other related conditions such as scleroderma, most have no clear cause of their Raynaud's. When no cause is identified we speak of having Raynaud's disease. Raynaud's disease is more common in women, usually begins in the 'teens or twenties, and often runs in families.

Raynaud's phenomenon in lupus may be mild and only be an inconvenience in the winter. Sometimes, however, it becomes more severe. The blood supply to the fingers is seriously diminished leading to painful sores on the finger tips or even loss of tissue at the tip of the finger.

Raynaud's can be treated. Staying warm during the winter with warm clothing and gloves is important. Since chemicals in cigarette smoke can cause spasm of the arteries, stopping smoking is a must. There are medications which can improve the circulation. The most successful are the so-called calcium channel blockers which are also used to treat high blood pressure and heart disease.

Antiphospholipid Syndrome

Another problem with circulation encountered by some people with SLE is the antiphospholipid antibody syndrome. This results in abnormal clotting of the blood. Antiphospholipid antibodies are antibodies directed against the fatty portion of the covering of the body's cells, most importantly, platelets. (Laboratory tests that are used to look for these antibodies are discussed in Chapter 3.)

Many people with antiphospholipid antibodies may never encounter any trouble as a result of having them. The antibodies may, however, cause blood clots. Sometimes these occur in the veins of the legs and lead to an inflammation (phlebitis). Other times the antiphospholipid antibodies may be associated with miscarriages. They cause the blood vessels in the placenta to close off with clots and not enough nourishment gets to the baby. When it is the arteries, rather than veins, where clotting occurs, strokes, heart attacks, or loss of blood supply to another part of the body can occur. Other problems that have been associated with antiphospholipid antibodies are low platelet counts, migraine headaches, and a bluish network-like discoloration of the skin called livedo reticularis.

Even when these antibodies are present, patients may not require treatment if there has not been evidence of clotting. A single aspirin a day may be used to reduce likelihood of clots forming. How to treat a first pregnancy in women with these antibodies is unclear, but in women with these antibodies who already have had miscarriages, blood thinning with a medication called heparin and careful monitoring of the baby have allowed many pregnancies to be concluded successfully. People who have had clots in their veins or arteries due to this syndrome are kept on the blood thinning medication coumadin indefinitely.

The Lungs

The most common effect of lupus on the lung is inflammation of the covering sac around the lung, pleuritis. This is similar to pericarditis, causing sharp chest pain which is increased with deep breaths. The diagnosis of pleuritis is made by the physician hearing a rubbing sound during breathing when the lungs are listened to with a stethoscope. At times fluid can develop in the space between the lungs and the chest wall. If a large amount of fluid collects it can be seen on an x-ray of the chest. The treatment of pleuritis is with nonsteroidal anti-inflammatory medications or with steroids.

Uncommonly, lupus can cause inflammation within the lung itself (pneumonitis). This leads to shortness of breath, and findings on chest x-ray that look like pneumonia. If that occurs, it is important for the physician to make sure that no infection has caused a similar problem or is complicating the lung problem caused by the lupus. This can often be accomplished by obtaining a sample of sputum (the thick mucous coughed up by the patient) and sending it to the laboratory for culture (a process that encourages any bacteria or germs to grow so they can be identified). One clue to the fact that the pneumonitis which is present is due to SLE is the observation that the disease is active elsewhere, for example, if the lupus skin rash or arthritis is flaring. Fever may accompany the pneumonitis of lupus or the pneumonia due to infection. Fever alone, therefore, does not help the physician decide the cause of inflammation in the lung. Sometimes repeated episodes of pneumonitis lead to fibrosis (scarring) of the lung with permanent loss of lung function.

A rare lung problem due to lupus is thickening of the blood vessels leading from the heart to the lung. This is called pulmonary hypertension and can cause heart failure of the right side of the heart (the side responsible for pumping blood into the lung). Shortness of breath on exertion may be the first sign of this problem.

Gastrointestinal Problems

Gastrointestinal (GI) problems in lupus can be caused by the disease and by medication used to treat the disease; the latter are more common.

When lupus itself causes GI symptoms, the complaint is usually of abdominal pain. The pain is often caused by

Lupus may be the cause of severe abdominal pain.

inflammation of the lining of the abdomen (peritonitis) or inflammation of the blood vessels to the intestines (vasculitis). The pain can occur intermittently and be relatively mild or be very severe and resemble an appendicitis or some other problem which requires surgery. At times nausea, vomiting, diarrhea, or bleeding may accompany the pain. Signs that lupus is active somewhere else in the body may be present. It can be difficult for doctors to tell when abdominal pain is from lupus and when it is from more common causes (inflamed gall bladder, etc.). At times, several different tests and even a trial period of treatment with steroids may be necessary to make the diagnosis of GI involvement due to lupus.

The medications most likely to cause stomach and bowel symptoms in people with lupus are the nonsteroidal anti-inflammatory drugs (NSAIDs). These include medications like aspirin (e.g. Ascriptin, Ecotrin); ibuprofen (e.g. Motrin, Advil, Nuprin) or naproxen (e.g. Naprosyn, Anaprox, Aleve) and many other medications used for arthritis. (See Table 3 and associated discussion in Chapter 5 for more about NSAIDS.) NSAIDs are commonly used in lupus not only to control arthritis but sometimes for pleuritis, pericarditis, fever and other manifestations. NSAIDs can cause upset stomach, pain, nausea or queasy sensation. Less commonly they can lead to ulcers or GI bleeding. There is not a clear relationship between symptoms and the serious side effects of ulcer pain and GI bleeding. The symptoms of NSAID use can be limited by giving the medication with food and by other medications used for indigestion.

NSAID ulcers are most common in people over 60 and in those taking steroids. The usual symptom of ulcers is pain below the end of the breastbone or under the ribs on the right side. The pain may awaken the person from sleep; it is typically relieved with food or antacids. The major complication of ulcers is bleeding. Bleeding may come to the attention of the doctor because of a drop in the patient's red blood cell count (measured by the hematocrit or hemoglobin) and is confirmed when the patient describes soft, black colored stools that resemble tar. If the bleeding is heavy, the patient may vomit blood and require emergency treatment.

Most people never have noticeable ulcers from NSAIDs even if they take these medications for many years. For people in whom ulcers are a serious risk such as those over 60, those also on steroids or those with a history of ulcer disease, a medicine called misoprostol (Cytotec) can be given along with NSAIDs to reduce the risk of developing an ulcer.

The Immune System

Some people with lupus develop swelling of their lymph nodes. The lymph nodes are bean-shaped glands that people usually only become aware of when they are enlarged. Lymph nodes are present all over the body but the

Pneumovax and flu shots are recommended.

places they are most commonly noticed by patients are under the arms, along the sides of the neck, and in the groin. When lymph node enlargement is the very first sign of SLE, it may be necessary to have a node biopsy performed (to have a surgeon obtain a small piece for a pathologist to examine). Actually there is nothing diagnostic about the appearance of the lymph node biopsy material in lupus. The biopsy is sometimes necessary because lymph nodes also enlarge in other diseases besides lupus and it is important to eliminate them as early as possible.

People with lupus who are on medications that suppress the immune system such as steroids, Imuran or Cytoxan are at increased risk of infection. Most of these are bacterial infections such as tuberculosis or infection with fungus. One viral infection that these immunosuppressive drugs may cause is shingles (known to doctors as herpes zoster). Shingles is caused by the same virus which causes chicken pox. It frequently starts with a localized pain, often on one side of the rib cage, next involves a red rash with tiny blisters in the area of the pain, and finally may lead to a long-lasting pain (post-herpetic neuralgia) which can continue for months or years. For a long time it was thought that there was no definite treatment for shingles, now it is believed that prompt treatment with an anti-viral drug (not a regular antibiotic!) can lessen the symptoms and prevent complications.

All infections in people with lupus need to be treated quickly. High fevers, more than 101 degrees Fahrenheit should prompt a call to your physician. It is also important for people with lupus to have all the appropriate vaccinations, especially the pneumonia vaccine, Pneumovax (currently recommended to be given every six years), and a yearly flu shot can be done safely in people with lupus and can be effective even though the patient is on moderate doses of prednisone (as much as 20mg/day).

Chapter 3. Laboratory Tests

Burton Zweiman, MD

Most physicians with a lot of experience in the care of lupus patients can make the diagnosis of systemic lupus erythematosus based upon certain findings when they take

> **No one laboratory test is diagnostic of lupus.**

a medical history and do a physical examination. Sometimes, early in lupus, however, these clinical clues are not well defined and the question arises whether there is a laboratory test that can diagnose lupus in all patients. Despite much research in this area, the answer is no. There is no one test which can do this.

The ANA Tests

The laboratory test performed most often as an aid in making a diagnosis of lupus is the immunofluorescence test which detects the presence of antinuclear antibody (ANA) in the blood. This is often simply called the ANA test. As Figure 1 shows, blood serum (the blood after the clot and the cells have been removed) drawn from a patient is reacted with human blood cells on a special plate. Because chemicals are added, the nuclei (the center portions) of these cells become visible under the microscope when they are attacked by antinuclear antibodies in the patient's serum. The ANA test is very helpful. Over ninety-

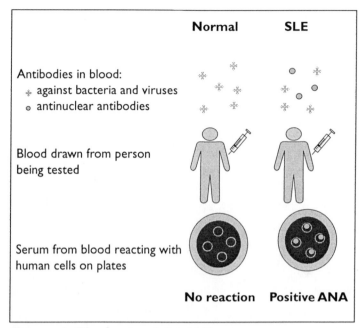

	Normal	SLE

Antibodies in blood:
  + against bacteria and viruses
  ○ antinuclear antibodies

Blood drawn from person being tested

Serum from blood reacting with human cells on plates

No reaction   **Positive ANA**

Figure 1. The basis of the ANA test

five percent of untreated lupus patients have high ANA levels in their blood. (A small number of individuals with SLE have a negative ANA. One group of these people have an unusual lupus disorder with a rash and an extreme sensitivity to sunlight.) For most people, not under intensive treatment, a negative result in several repeated ANA tests, performed in a good laboratory, is strong evidence against the diagnosis of systemic lupus erythematosus.

The ANA test is not specific for lupus. This means the ANA can be positive in other diseases, including some disorders with symptoms similar to lupus. (See Table 2.) Sometimes this lack of specificity leads to confusion and a diagnosis of lupus may be made in error just because the ANA is positive. Although ANA levels in the blood are generally higher in untreated lupus patients than in patients with other diseases, this is not always so. A diagnosis of lupus, therefore, cannot be made only on the basis of a high ANA.

Table 2. PERCENTAGE OF POSITIVE ANA TESTS AMONG THOSE WITH CONDITIONS SOMETIMES CONFUSED WITH LUPUS

CONDITION	POSITIVE ANA
Systemic lupus erythematosus	95% or more
Scleroderma	70% to 90%
Sjogren's syndrome	60% to 80%
Rheumatoid arthritis	about 40%
Polymyositis	10% to 50%
Mixed connective tissue disease	80% to 90%
Drug induced lupus	variable %'s
Good health	less than 4%*

* *Increases with age*

Individual ANA Antibodies

Much research has been done to expand and refine the ANA test in order to find a test that is more specific for lupus. To understand this effort, it is helpful to know that the ANA is actually a group of antibodies directed against different parts of the body's cells. Antibodies are substances our bodies normally make against things considered "foreign", like bacteria. In that way, antibodies can protect us from getting certain infections. Normally we make little or no autoantibodies, antibodies directed against our own cells. A few people, however, are predisposed to make such autoantibodies, including antinuclear antibodies directed at the nucleus of the cell. Almost all of the cells in our body have a central part called the nucleus. This holds most of the genetic material which we inherit and pass on to our children. Contained in this genetic material are instructions telling the rest of the cell how to function. It is not yet known why the nuclear material inside the cell becomes a target for autoantibodies which circulate in the blood. In the laboratory, cells are "opened up" and, with special procedures, antibodies against different parts can be detected individually. Some of these individual antinuclear antibodies are very specific for the diagnosis of lupus:

1. *Anti-ds (double-stranded) DNA antibodies.* These antibodies react to DNA, the material which makes up the genes found in cells. Double-stranded DNA also plays a key role in the growth and multiplication of these cells. Increasing blood levels of anti-ds antibodies are found in about 70% of lupus patients, and found very infrequently in other disorders. However, the dsDNA used in the test must be prepared very carefully so that it does not contain single stranded DNA. Antibodies against this single stranded DNA are commonly found in disorders other than lupus, and can confuse the results of the test. Anti-ds DNA antibodies are more commonly found in lupus patients whose disease is active, particularly if the disease involves the kidneys or the central nervous system.

2. *Anti-Sm (Smith) antibodies.* These antibodies are named after the patient in whom they were first found. They react with another part of the cell nucleus, and are found in about 30% of lupus patients. Anti-Sm antibodies are found very rarely in disorders other than lupus.

3. *Anti-Ro (or SS-A) antibodies.* These are found in some lupus patients, particularly some with a sun sensitive rash. If a pregnant lupus patient has anti-Ro antibodies, it is more likely that her baby will have a certain type of congenital heart disorder, although this occurs in only a small percentage of cases. Anti-Ro antibodies are also found in a disorder called Sjogren's syndrome (causing, among other things a dry mouth and dry eyes). Sometimes Sjogren's syndrome occurs with lupus.

4. *Antihistone antibodies.* These antibodies are found in the blood of many lupus patients and are directed against a protein which is frequently attached to the DNA within the cell nucleus. Similar antihistone antibodies are also found in the blood of some people who have high levels of ANA caused by taking certain medications.

5. *Anti-RNP (ribonucleoprotein) antibodies.* These antibodies occur commonly in lupus and some other disorders. Certain individuals, mainly women, develop a group of symptoms that do not point strongly to lupus or to one of the other connective tissue inflammatory diseases (like rheumatoid arthritis or scleroderma), but rather to a combination of several of these diseases. This

combination has been called "mixed connective tissue disease" or "overlap syndrome".

Other Antibody Tests

In some individuals with lupus, there are abnormal blood proteins that appear to be antibodies against something on the surface of platelets. Platelets are particles in the blood involved in normal blood clotting. Sometimes these abnormal antibodies prolong blood clotting and are detected by blood clotting tests. (Then they are referred to as a lupus anticoagulant). Sometimes they are detected by a particular antibody test which detects anticardiolipin antibodies. Some of the people with these abnormal proteins develop what is known as the antiphospholipid syndrome. (For more about this syndrome, see Chapter 2.) They have a tendency to develop clots in their veins and arteries and the women may have miscarriages. (See Chapter 18 on Lupus and Pregnancy.) Of interest, these antibodies can also result in a false positive screening blood test for syphilis. An individual with such antibodies who is tested for syphilis, as when applying for a marriage license, may be told that the test is positive even though he or she does not in fact have syphilis. Fortunately, there are now additional tests that distinguish between "true" and "false" positive tests for syphilis.

Several other antibody tests are often performed when attempting to make a diagnosis of lupus because they help to tell the difference between lupus and other diseases. Antiscleroderma 70 (anti-Scl-70) antibodies are found in some people with one form of scleroderma. Anticentromere antibodies are commonly found in another form of scleroderma. Anti-PM 1 and anti-Jo-1 antibodies are found in polymyositis. Rheumatoid factor is found in a great majority of people with rheumatoid arthritis, a condition which not uncommonly is confused with lupus. Rheumatoid factor may also be found in the blood of about 20% of lupus patients, and in a number of other disorders.

Other Laboratory Tests

The levels of certain proteins in the blood called complement components, may be low in lupus patients particularly when the disease is active. Complement can be thought of as part of the ammunition of the immune system. When the disease is active, more ammunition is expended to fight it off and the body's complement supply runs low. Low complement levels are not very helpful in diagnosing lupus, however, because low levels can be found in other diseases as well and some people are born with low complement levels. Complement levels are useful both in following the activity of the disease and the response to treatment of individual patients. The erythrocyte sedimentation rate (ESR) is the rate at which red blood cells settle in a test tube. It is also used as a measure of inflammation in lupus and many other conditions. Unfortunately, this simple, inexpensive test is not a very reliable measure of whether lupus has become

Some antibody tests help distinguish lupus from similar diseases.

inactive.

There are many laboratory tests which can help to detect whether specific organ systems are affected by lupus. The results of these tests can be very valuable in the care of the individual lupus patient. These will be discussed in other chapters. However, several examples are described briefly here.

Kidney involvement in lupus can be suspected by examining individual urine specimens. Such involvement can also be determined by measuring the amount of protein found in the urine during a 24 hour period. The 24 hour urine collection can also be used to find out if there is any decrease in the filtering function of the kidneys. In certain situations it may be necessary to perform a kidney biopsy to find out what type of involvement of the kidney is present. This involves inserting a needle through the back which has been made numb by a local anesthetic. (See Chapter 7 for more about lupus and the kidney).

Involvement of the central nervous system occurs commonly in lupus, but is often difficult to diagnose. A spinal tap to collect some of the cerebrospinal fluid (fluid which is present around the spinal cord and the brain) is sometimes helpful in this regard. This fluid is abnormal in about 50% of patients with the central nervous system involvement of lupus. Computerized axial tomography (CAT scans) and magnetic resonance imaging (MRI) signals are now also being used to help diagnose involvement of the nervous system in lupus. (More about nervous system involvement and its diagnosis in Chapters 8 and 9.)

A complete blood count (CBC) measures the level

of red cells, white cells and platelets in the blood and is commonly ordered in lupus patients. Anemia, or a low red blood count, is frequently the result of disease activity. Levels of white blood cells (leukocytes), and platelets (small blood particles which are part of the clotting mechanism) may also be reduced in active lupus. This happens so often that these particular abnormal findings are considered one of the criteria on which the diagnosis of lupus is based. (See Table 1 and Chapter 12.)

Summary

There is no test which is as specific for lupus as we would like. If a person has repeated normal results using current, very sensitive ANA blood tests, this is very strong evidence against a diagnosis of lupus. Results obtained from a group of available antibody tests can help the experienced physician distinguish lupus from other conditions with similar symptoms. One antibody test indicates a tendency people with lupus, and others, have to form blood clots and has special implications in pregnancy. Other tests help to measure the response to treatment in lupus and can help to determine whether or not disease activity is increasing. Intensive research is leading to new tests of the immune system. Hopefully, these will lead to easier diagnoses and improved treatment.

Chapter 4. Genetics

Raphael J. DeHoratius, MD

The most frequently asked question about lupus is, "Is lupus inherited?" The answer to this question is both "yes" and "no"! Genes, those parts of our individual make-up that we inherit from our parents, are important in the development of lupus, but the answer is much more complicated than a simple "yes". Estimates are that from four to six or more genes must be

> **Is lupus inherited? Answer: "Yes" and "No".**

combined for a person to inherit a susceptibility to acquire lupus. It is nearly impossible to inherit all the genes necessary to develop lupus from a single parent, since an individual's genes come from both

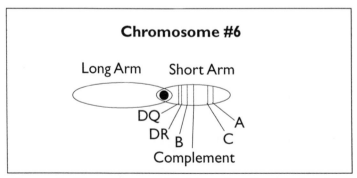

Figure 2. Chromosome #6. Lines leading to the short arm point to the corresponding HLA regions (A,B,C,DR,DQ) and to the region where complement is located.

parents. This is one very important reason why it is unusual for lupus to occur in multiple generations of a family. If only some of the lupus genes are inherited, a person may not have lupus but may test positive for some of the immunologic tests, such as the antinuclear antibody (ANA). A positive ANA occurs in up to one third of healthy family members of lupus patients.

Genetic information is coded in chromosomes which are located in humans in a tiny part of the center (nucleus) of each cell. Humans have 46 chromosomes, each of which is made up of thousands of genes. Each chromosome is divided into a long and short arm with a small center portion called the centromere. Many of the important genes in systemic lupus erythematosus are located on the short arm of chromosome #6.

The genes on chromosome #6 have many complex functions. Some regulate complement components (proteins important in acute and chronic inflammation and in the formation of immune complexes). When these complement components are missing, a milder form of lupus, which usually lacks kidney involvement, may develop. Complement genes are important but they are not the whole story in the development of this form of lupus. For example, many susceptible individuals who lack these genes for complement never develop lupus at all.

Other important areas on the short arm of chromosome #6 are the HLA (human leukocyte antigen) regions. They are located near the area for complement genes. These HLA areas have been very thoroughly studied since they are used to match donors genetically to recipients for organ transplants. HLA areas include different regions called HLA-A, HLA-B, HLA-C, HLA-DR, HLA-DQ. In each of these regions, each individual inherits different genes which are designated by numbers. In lupus patients there is an increased frequency of the HLA genes known as A1, B8, DR2, DR3 and DQ1.

Associations between genes and diseases such as lupus are established by comparing lupus patients to a normal or "control" population. Particular HLA markers found in white lupus patients (on whom the majority of studies have focused) have not been shown to be identical in black patients or Japanese patients with lupus. The reasons for these differences are not entirely clear. There may be other, as yet unknown, genes or there may also be important genes on other chromosomes which play a part in making a person susceptible to developing lupus. These may include the genes that control for complement receptors or the genes that control for immunoglobulin production (the proteins that fight infection).

The newest research methods now being used to study genetics come from the field of molecular biology. They are redefining the way in which we look at the genetics of disease. When methods of molecular biology are used to study the HLA system in various diseases, we are finding that what we used to think was a specific HLA gene is, in reality, a large group of very slightly different genes. This new knowledge should lead to new important findings, both in genetics and in lupus.

Another way of studying the genetics of lupus is by looking at families in which lupus occurs in more than one member. Familial cases are reported in approximately 10% of the lupus population. The most thoroughly studied family association is between twins. If one of a pair of identical twins (twins with exactly the same genes) has lupus, the other will develop it more than two thirds (69%) of the time. If a fraternal or non-identical twin (a twin with genes no more similar to his twin than to any other brother or sister) has lupus, the other twin has only a 5% chance of developing it. It is obvious that genetics are important, since the frequency of developing lupus is so much higher in identical *twins* than in fraternal twins when one of the twins already has lupus. Genetic factors cannot be the only answers, however, or susceptible identical twins would both develop lupus 100% of the time. Environmental factors, therefore, must also be important. It appears that some people are genetically predisposed to develop lupus but then must be exposed to the proper environmental triggers in order to have the disease.

If one identical twin has lupus, the other is likely to have it too.

In summary, heredity is involved in the development of lupus but it is rare to have more than one family member who has lupus. Much is known about the genetics of lupus, yet even more needs to be discovered. It is only through careful family studies using very modern scientific techniques (molecular biology) that the answer to the genetic riddle of sys-

temic lupus erythematosus and the relationship between heredity and environment will be solved.

Chapter 5. Disease Management

Peter Callegari, MD

One of the most important parts of a long-term treatment program for patients with lupus is the development of a sense of trust and open communication between physician and patient. (More about this in Chapter 20.) Lupus patients are the best source of information about the pattern of their own disease activity. Both the physician and patient should be alert to changes in symptoms. Sometimes, the development of mild symptoms may suggest that the illness is becoming more active. Vague symptoms such as malaise (a general feeling of being unwell), poor appetite, and increased fatigue are often associated with a flare-up of lupus but may also be due to other causes. Working together, the patient and the physician can best determine the cause of such symptoms so appropriate treatment can be started. Such teamwork should reduce unnecessary hospitalization, testing, expense, and anxiety.

Exercise

Most lupus patients are young women who expect – and are expected by others – to lead active vigorous lives. Thus it is important that families, as well as patients, understand the limitations that lupus may impose. An active, full life is a goal that can be reached, but everyone involved must accept the fact that periods of fatigue and depression (Discussed in Chapter 10.) may occur even in mild cases. Patients often need time to themselves for both physical and emotional rest. At other times, patients may feel alone and isolated by their disease.

Rest and exercise must be balanced.

Then they can benefit from participation in a lupus support group. (See Chapter 19.) A balance between exercise and rest is also desirable. Flare-ups of disease activity call for increased rest, including daytime naps. Too much rest, though, can cause loss of muscle mass and muscle tone resulting in weakness, fatigue, further reduction in activity and depression. As the disease comes under control, a regularly scheduled exercise program should be undertaken to increase strength, endurance and muscle tone. A physical therapist or another health care professional can often be helpful in teaching the patient a proper exercise program. (See Chapter 16 for more about exercise.)

Diet

Nutrition is an important aspect of maintaining health and treating any chronic illness. Nutrition becomes particularly important in SLE since both the illness and medications used to treat it can cause changes in appetite and weight. A balanced diet is the most appropriate one. There is no definite scientific proof that a special diet is harmful or helpful in lupus. However, there have been reports of lupus starting up or flaring when alfalfa seeds or sprouts were eaten. Conversely, there have been suggestions that certain polyunsaturated fatty acids, such as are found in fish oil, might have a beneficial effect on lupus. Vitamin supplements are not necessary in most cases. It is important to maintain an adequate calcium intake. This can be done through eating calcium containing foods or taking calcium supplements (a relatively inexpensive supplement is provided by Tums-type antacids.) Maintenance of ideal weight is desirable but may be difficult for patients taking medicines like corticosteroids. Control of weight is particularly important in people with arthritis, high blood pressure, diabetes and those with kidney disease. A regular program of moderate exercise can be very useful in a weight control program.

Lupus patients with special needs or problems may require special diets. Medications, such as corticosteroids, or conditions like hypertension can make it necessary to restrict salt intake, monitor cholesterol levels and limit calories.

Medications

When lupus is not active, there may be no need for medications. Rest, an exercise program, a balanced diet, and avoidance of the sun may be all that is necessary. When lupus is active and drug treatment is

There is no one right way to treat lupus.

needed, a variety of medications are available. There is no one right way to treat lupus. Drug treatment will vary depending upon the various effects of the disease as well as with the doctor's training and previous experience using the various medications.

Nonsteroidal anti-inflammatory drugs (NSAIDS)

When medication is needed, many doctors turn first to the NSAIDs. These agents are the most commonly used medicines to treat SLE. There are many NSAIDs on the market. Some of the most widely used are listed in Table 3 which gives the trade or common name and the generic name. NSAIDs are all distant relatives of aspirin, sharing similar benefits and similar side effects. They all relieve pain as well as inflammation. NSAIDs can be used to control fever, as well as arthritis and inflammation elsewhere (pericarditis, pleuritis, etc.). Most NSAIDs are given two or three times daily with meals. All can irritate the stomach and can (rarely) lead to ulcers. Effects on the digestive system include heartburn, indigestion, stomach and abdominal pain, nausea, vomiting and bleeding from the stomach. NSAIDs can cause fluid retention and problems with the functioning of the kidneys. They should be used with caution in lupus patients who have high blood pressure kidney disease or heart failure. Like aspirin, other NSAIDs can make it harder for blood to clot and for bleeding to stop. No one NSAID is better to treat lupus than any other. Different NSAIDs react differently in any one patient. If one NSAID is not well tolerated or is ineffective, it is usual to try another before giving up on this category of drugs.

Aspirin itself can be used as an NSAID but it also has a role in the treatment of blood clotting. It does this by interfering with the way our platelets work.

Table 3. SOME COMMONLY PRESCRIBED NSAIDS*

TRADE NAME	GENERIC NAME
Ansaid	flubiprofen
Aspirin	acetylsalicylic acid
Clinoril	sulindac
Daypro	oxaprozin
Feldene	piroxicam
Indocin	indomethacin
Lodine	etodolac
Motrin	ibuprofen
Nalfon	fenoprofen
Naprosyn	naproxen
Orudis	ketoprofen
Oruvail	ketoprofen
Relafen	nabumetone
Tolectin	tolmetin
Trilisate	magnesium/choline salicylate
Voltaren	diclofenac

* There are many other NSAIDs. Your pharmacist or doctor can tell you if a medicine not on this list is an NSAID.

Platelets are cell pieces in our blood that help to "plug" up leaks in our blood vessels which cause us to bleed. In some cases of SLE, the body makes inappropriate blood clots. (See Chapter 12 on lupus and the blood.) In these people, aspirin in very low does, may prevent such clots from forming.

Aspirin has always been available "over the counter" (without a doctor's prescription). In recent years, in the United States, several other NSAIDs have also become available in this way. These include ibuprofen (Advil, Nuprin, Motrin IB), naproxen (Aleve), and ketoprofen (Orudis KT). It is very important for patients taking NSAIDs which have been prescribed by their doctors to be aware that these "over the counter" medications are similar. To avoid NSAID overdose and to minimize side effects or interference of one drug with another, patients should check with their physicians before treating themselves with these readily available medicines.

Antimalarial medications

The antimalarial drugs are so-called because they were originally used to treat malaria. These drugs have proven to be very useful in treating some of the problems of lupus. The antimalarials include hydroxychloroquine (Plaquenil), quinacrine (Atabrine) and chloroquine (Aralen). The arthritis and skin disease of lupus respond especially well to antimalarial drugs. Antimalarial medications are usually slow acting and may not take effect for weeks or months. Some patients who do not benefit from one antimalarial drug will respond well to another. Occasional patients with sun-induced rashes do well with antimalarial treatment during spring and summer and are able to discontinue it in the winter.

Nausea, loss of appetite, and indigestion are common in many patients begun on a full dose of an antimalarial. A temporary reduction in dose or half of a regular dose given twice daily may help to avoid these problems. Occasionally, increased skin pigmentation (darkening of the skin, "freckling" or brown spots) may develop in a patient on an antimalarial. This is usually reversible and the skin lightens after the antimalarial is stopped.

The most serious (although extremely rare) potential side effects of antimalarial medications involve the eye. All lupus patients treated with these medicines should be examined every six to twelve months by an ophthalmologist. The risk of permanent damage to the retina (the light sensitive layer of the eye) is very low but is real. This risk is related to the quantity of antimalarials taken and by keeping the dose low, it can be minimized. Regular retinal examinations by an ophthalmologist, who is familiar with antimalarial

Special eye exams are essential when taking antimalarial drugs.

drugs and with lupus, can alert the physician and patient to any problems. Blurred vision may also occur early in the course of treatment with any of the antimalarial medications. This is due to deposit of the drug in the cornea (the transparent window in the front of the eye). The effect on vision is temporary and usually disappears as the drug is continued. Because of possible effects on the eye, a full discussion of the benefits and risks of antimalarial medications is advisable before treatment with these drugs is begun.

Corticosteroids

Corticosteroids (prednisone, prednisolone, methylprednisolone or Medrol) are cortisone-like medications used to treat the more severe complications of lupus such as central nervous system and kidney disorders. Corticosteroids are substances normally found in the body. Every person makes a daily supply and, in times of severe illness or stress, the normal amount is increased. When prescribed for lupus, these medications can have powerful positive effects on the disease. They also have many powerful unwanted side effects, however. Because of this, doctors always try to keep the dose of corticosteroids as low as possible and to discontinue them whenever possible.

For patients who do need corticosteroids from time to time, an "aggressive-conservative" approach is thought to be best. This calls for treating a flare-up with relatively high doses (aggressive) of prednisone, a type of steroid, but for as short a period as possible (conservative). The "aggressive" part of this approach has led to the increasing rate of survival of lupus patients in recent years as physicians have learned to use corticosteroids more effectively. The "conservative" is used because of the well-known side effects of corticosteroid treatment. The dosage of prednisone varies, since each patient responds individually. Despite the appearance of side effects, treatment must be continued until the flare is under control. Studies have shown that, unfortunately, about 30% of patients do not take medication as prescribed.

Corticosteroids are prescribed differently at different stages of illness. When the patient is very ill with lupus, high doses are prescribed, often in divided doses (two or three times a day). When the disease is less active, the daily dose can be consolidated and gradually reduced. When lupus is controlled, the drug can often be completely stopped or maintained at a low dose. Some people can be maintained on an alternate day (every-other-day) dose which is believed to reduce side effects. On rare occasions, usually when lupus causes very serious illness, "pulse" or "bolus" corticosteroids are used. Very high doses are given very rapidly, often by vein. Intravenous pulse therapy is now being widely used with very promising results.

It is important to remember never to stop corticosteroids unless instructed how to do so by your physician! After being taken for a while, these medications replace the corticosteroids which your body itself makes. Your body then senses that its work is not needed and temporarily shuts down its "factory", making no corticosteroids on its own. If you then abruptly stop taking steroid medication, your body has no ability to

Never stop steroids without your doctor's knowledge.

deal with stress by increasing its own supply of this vital substance. Life threatening shock can result. If you are on corticosteroid medication for a long period of time, it is a wise practice to wear a Medi-Alert bracelet or necklace which records this fact. Then, if you ever have a medical emergency and are unable to communicate, the medallion will inform doctors that you take corticosteroids and they will not mistakenly discontinue them.

Patients react to corticosteroids in different ways. Some experience marked side effects fairly soon on very small doses, and others can take fairly high doses for weeks without trouble. Some experience emotional disturbances – feelings of agitation and depression, difficulty sleeping, unaccustomed dreaming, and a sense that they are losing control. More commonly, people experience increased appetite and feel full of nervous energy, "edgy," or "wired," as if they are taking too much caffeine.

There are many long-term problems also believed to be caused by taking corticosteroids. Osteoporosis (thinning of the bones) is clearly made worse by these drugs. The use of supplementary calcium is recommended to help prevent bone loss. (Other treatment for osteoporosis is available and is recommended for each person individually.) Cataracts (clouding of the lenses of the eye) are also caused by corticosteroids. (See Chapter 11 on the eye.) Avascular necrosis (localized death of bone tissue) can occur in patients with lupus, usually those on steroids. (Discussed in full in Chapter 13.) Stunting of the growth in a child or adolescent is also a possibility since young bones mature rapidly on these medications. Stomach ulcers, high blood pressure, elevated cholesterol and atherosclerosis (hardening of the arteries which can lead to heart disease) are also possible side-effects. All are believed to be related to the total dose of corticosteroids. This supports the use of as little corticosteroid treatment as possible over the years.

Immunosuppressive Drugs

Immunosuppressive drugs were first developed to treat cancer. They work, in part, because they reduce the activity of the patient's immune system. Therapy with these drugs such as azathioprine (Imuran), cyclophosphamide (Cytoxan), and chlorambucil (Leukeran) is used in those patients with the most severe disease. These drugs are very effective. They can often control the disease enough to allow the dose of corticosteroids to be lowered. This is often

Some drugs call for very close monitoring by the physician.

referred as a "steroid sparing" benefit of these medications. They can be given as a daily dose by mouth or can be given once monthly or less often as a medicine in the vein. Patients taking these drugs must have frequent blood counts since all of them can affect the bone marrow, the place where blood cells are made. By decreasing the platelets, they may increase the chance of bleeding. By lowering the white blood cells, they may lower the body's defenses against infection. By decreasing red blood cells and causing anemia, they may cause fatigue and heart failure. These drugs can also cause abnormalities in a developing fetus and are not recommended for women who may become pregnant. Another real concern with these drugs is the remote possibility that they might cause cancer. Rare cases of leukemia and other malignancies have been reported in patients taking these drugs for an extended period.

Methotrexate (Rheumatrex), a drug similar to this

cytotoxic group, is widely used to treat rheumatoid arthritis and is also being used in SLE. Blood counts must also be tested regularly in people on methotrexate. Studies of the liver are also needed since methotrexate taken for a long time can sometimes damage that organ.

All of the drugs in this group require very careful follow-up by the doctor. They are safest when administered by a physician who uses them frequently and has a good understanding of both all of their side effects and potential benefits.

Other Treatments

Special problems which occur in SLE may require uncommon treatments and medications. These are discussed briefly below.

Pheresis is a method of removing parts of the blood from the body. In people with lupus, plasmapheresis (removal of plasma, the liquid part of the blood which contains no blood cells) can temporarily eliminate the antibodies which damage the skin, the kidney etc. By taking away these antibodies, the lupus can sometimes be controlled until other medicines begin to work. Plasmapheresis is very expensive and is effective for only a short time. It is usually reserved for those cases of lupus in which the illness is moving ahead rapidly.

Cyclosporine is a medication derived from a fungus which has very powerful effects on the immune system. It has been used to treat some people who cannot get relief from the standard medications. It is particularly difficult to use in lupus patients, however, because it can cause high blood pressure and worsen kidney function, two problems which are common in lupus.

Dapsone is an antibiotic used to treat leprosy. It has also proven to be a very effective medication in the treatment of bullous (blistering) lupus erythematosus. Dapsone has also been used to treat vasculitis. Dapsone can cause sudden anemia, low numbers of red blood cells, and blood counts must be checked regularly.

Danazol is a steroid but is not closely related to cortisone or the other corticosteroids. It is most like the male hormones, the androgens. Danazol is sometimes used to treat very low platelet counts and other manifestations of SLE. Among its side effects are increased irritability and, in women, the growth of facial hair and deepening of the voice.

New Agents and The Future

There is a real need for new treatments for lupus which are more effective and which are safer. There are a number of treatments in development and more will become available as we continue to study and understand this illness. Some of the most promising new research agents are known as biologicals. This is a family of treatments made in the laboratory from the body's own materials or from material designed to imitate these materials. Most attempt to improve lupus by removing or blocking inflammation signals. Some block the abnormal antibodies made by lupus patients.

DHEA (dehydroepiandrosterone) is a naturally occurring hormone which, in early studies, has shown some promise in the treatment of lupus arthritis and the loss of energy associated with lupus. There is also the suggestion that DHEA may allow lupus patients to decrease their steroid dosage. Large, controlled studies of DHEA are currently going on. If these also demonstrate effectiveness, the drug will be submitted for Food and Drug Administration approval for use in lupus.

Intravenous gamma globulin (IVIG) has also been used to treat some of the problems caused by SLE, including the low platelet counts and the abnormal blood clotting that sometimes occur. Generally IVIG is given by vein for several days in a row. The treatment is temporary and can be quite expensive.

Research is also underway into using natural diet supplements to treat SLE. Newer agents to treat joint inflammation are also appearing. And research into SLE itself is progressing so that, in the future, as we further understand it, we may be able to fit the treatment for each individual.

Summary

Although a cure for lupus is not yet available, management of the disease continues to improve. An understanding of lupus on the part of the patient and an open, comfortable relationship between patient and physician is essential to good long-term care. The patient's family must also be informed about lupus and be aware of how it might affect the patient. A variety of medications are used to treat lupus patients. The types and amount of medicine taken will vary according to the activity of the lupus.

Chapter 6. The Skin

Guy F. Webster, MD, PhD

No manifestations of lupus are so noticeable or potentially disfiguring as those which affect the skin. Two different settings in which skin disease appears in lupus are chronic cutaneous lupus, sometimes referred to as discoid lupus erythematosus (DLE), and systemic lupus erythematosus (SLE). Skin changes which occur in DLE are chiefly of the discoid variety described below. Those which occur in SLE are of many different kinds.

> **If you are tanning, you are not well enough protected from the sun.**

Photosensitivity (a tendency to overreact to sunlight) is common to both SLE and DLE. It can make both conditions worse and avoidance of sun is an important part of the treatment of both. Both the "sunburn" wavelengths (ultraviolet B, 290 to 320 nm) and the "tanning" wavelengths (ultraviolet A, 320 to 400 nm) can trigger flares. Patients with lupus should avoid excessive sun exposure by confining outdoor activities to the morning and late afternoon, by wearing protective clothing and by the conscientious use of sunscreens that block both ultraviolet A and B. Such sunscreens are those with a sun protective factor (SPF) of 15 or greater. A good rule of thumb is that if you are getting tanned, you are not well enough protected.

Chronic cutaneous lupus or DLE is a form of lupus which is almost entirely limited to the skin. Patients with this condition have red, scaly patches on the skin, especially over the face, scalp and upper back. When these heal after being present for only a short time, the skin again appears normal. When they are present for a long time, however, they can cause permanent scarring of the skin. The skin in the affected patches gets thinner, becomes pale, and loses its hair and sweat glands. Permanent, patchy, baldness can result. Openings in the skin (actually tiny sacs or follicles), out of which hair once grew, become prominent and can give the affected areas a pigskin-like appearance. Patients with chronic cutaneous lupus have very little chance of developing systemic lupus erythematosus. Only about ten percent have a positive ANA and a small proportion of this group eventually go on to develop systemic disease.

Chronic cutaneous lupus does not usually progress to SLE.

There are two major aspects of the treatment of DLE. Avoidance of the sun is paramount. About half of patients with DLE have disease which will flare when they are exposed to the sun. The second aspect of the treatment of DLE involves the use of medications designed to decrease inflammation or to turn off the disease process. If the affected skin is limited to a few small sized skin areas, corticosteroid creams and ointments or injections into the skin are safe and effective. Because one injection into an area of discoid rash typically is effective for three to four weeks and delivers the medication right into the area of the disease, many dermatologists prefer to use injections rather than creams or ointments. When the skin involvement is more extensive, short courses of steroids by mouth (prednisone, Medrol, etc.) may be used. Sometimes it may also be useful to treat widespread skin disease with antimalarial drugs (hydroxychloroquine, chloroquine). Rarely, immunosuppressive drugs (azathioprine, cyclophosphamide, etc.) may be needed for particularly resistant disease.

The systemic form of lupus, SLE, has several possible skin manifestations. The classic malar or "butterfly" rash on the nose and cheeks is the one that is most typically associated with lupus, but there are many others. The butterfly rash is often difficult to diagnose as a sign of lupus with certainty. Other very common skin conditions affecting the central part of the face, such as rosacea and seborrheic dermatitis, are easily confused with the classic lupus rash. To further complicate matters, patients who have lupus may have these other conditions as well. Rosacea, which commonly causes flushing and prominent blood vessels of the face is often worsened by corticosteroids. This may cause the patient with lupus who also has rosacea to appear to have a flare of his or her facial lupus in spite of the improvement of lupus elsewhere.

Other skin signs of SLE include the results of inflammation of blood vessels (vasculitis) that may appear as hives (urticaria) or purple-red spots (purpura), a purplish network patterned rash (livedo reticularis), or the presence of small groups of tiny blood vessels (telangiectasia) on the face, chest and hands. Loss of scalp hair (alopecia) and painless raw areas (ulcers) of the mucous membranes (the moist coverings or linings) of the mouth, the eyes, the vagina and the penis may occur. Although all forms of SLE may be worsened by sun exposure, the form of lupus called "subacute cutaneous lupus" is particularly sensitive to ultraviolet light. The rash in this form of lupus often appears as slightly scaly skin changes in a ring-like shape. It is most commonly found in areas of the skin that are commonly exposed to the sun such as the arms, upper back, and upper chest.

SLE can cause many skin changes besides the "butterfly" rash

A skin biopsy often provides important evidence to assist in the diagnosis of lupus. The skin is made numb with an injection of local anesthetic, then a very small piece of skin with the underlying connective tissue, fat, and muscle is removed. Typically, two kinds of analysis are done on the biopsy specimen. In the first, the sample is stained with various dyes that allow the pathologist to identify the type of damage which has taken place. In the second, known as immunofluorescence, antibodies that may have deposited on the skin are identified. In lupus, these antibodies are found in a band between the upper and lower layers of the skin, a positive "band" test. The band test is of special interest since it may be positive even in a patient with no visible skin changes.

A skin biopsy may be useful even when no rash is obvious.

Because lupus often shows itself first as a skin disease, dermatologists have always played an important role in developing knowledge about the disease. When a case suspected of being lupus proves to be difficult to diagnose, it is often helpful to consult a dermatologist.

Chapter 7. The Kidney

Louis J. Riley, Jr., MD and
Alan G. Wasserstein, MD

The kidney plays a role in carrying out several major tasks for the body. By forming about two quarts

---

Table 4. KIDNEY FUNCTIONS

Filter and clean blood
Eliminate extra fluid
Balance body chemicals
Help control blood pressure
Make vitamin D to build bone
Raise red blood cell count

---

of urine daily, the kidneys contribute to ridding the body of its wastes and controlling the amount of essential fluids and chemicals. As a result of the fluid and chemical control, blood pressure is regulated. The kidney also manufactures two important chemicals – an active form of vitamin D which helps to control calcium for building bones and a hormone called erythropoietin which stimulates the bone marrow to make red blood cells.

Lupus does not always affect the kidney, but when it does, kidney disease may be one of the lupus patient's most significant health problems. Kidney problems in lupus are due to the production of abnormal autoantibodies. These antibodies are directed against the patient's own tissue, for example, against DNA, the genetic material which is found in most of the body's cells, including those which make up the kidney. The formation of immune complexes (combinations of these antibodies joining with normal body substances) sets up an inflammatory reaction in the kidney.

Several serious kidney disorders can result. Minor abnormalities in urine or blood test results often provide the clues that damage to the kidneys exists. Such abnormalities include excessive amounts of protein in the urine, red blood cells in the urine, or a rise in the serum creatinine (a waste product which is

---

Table 5. KIDNEY DISEASE TREATMENT

Control of diet and fluids
Medications to control:
    Blood pressure
    Fluid balance
    Red blood cell count
    Calcium and phosphate
    Activity of the lupus
Dialysis
    Peritoneal dialysis
    Hemodialysis
Kidney transplantation

---

measured in the blood). The damaged kidney sometimes leaks large amounts of protein, a condition called the nephrotic syndrome. As part of this syndrome, the ability of the kidneys to remove salt and water from the body is impaired. Excess fluid collects in the legs and abdomen and around the eyes, causing discomfort and inconvenience. Patients may find that their clothes or shoes have become too tight to wear. Diuretics ("water pills") are usually prescribed to help eliminate the excess fluid by increasing urination.

If kidney damage caused by lupus is diagnosed and treated early, the treatment is usually most effective. A kidney biopsy is the best way to determine the extent of disease and the need for treatment. A biopsy is done with the patient lying on his or her side after the kidneys have been precisely located by means of ultra-sound or a CAT scan. The patient is awake and only a local anesthetic is required. A tiny cylinder of kidney tissue is withdrawn with a special needle. This tissue is examined under a microscope so details of the kidney structure can be examined. Since there is a risk of bleeding from the kidney, the patient must stay in the hospital for observation for several hours or overnight following the biopsy.

A treatment plan is developed on the basis of information obtained from the biopsy sample. Mild abnormalities, present in almost all lupus patients, even those with no other clinical or laboratory evidence of kidney involvement, require no treatment. More serious disease may require diet and fluid management to reduce protein and water intake, diuretics and other medications to lower blood pressure and control calcium and phosphate balance, and drugs aimed at decreasing the activity of the lupus itself.

To control lupus activity, corticosteroids, such as prednisone, have been the basis of treatment for many years. Their use may result in some improvement in lupus kidney disease, but the improvement is not as long lasting as we would like. A significant modern advance in the treatment of lupus-related kidney disease has been the use of drugs to suppress the immune system, for example, Cytoxan (cyclophosphamide). Such drugs reduce the production of antibodies which cause inflammation. Cytoxan is usually given in combination with prednisone. In many cases it has led to clear improvement in lupus kidney disease. This has been demonstrated by observing improvement in biopsy specimens, reduction in the amount of protein in the urine, and improvement in the kidney's ability to remove wastes. Cytoxan is a toxic drug, however, which has many side effects. These include a decrease in the white blood cell count which makes a patient more susceptible to bacterial and other infections. It can also cause bleeding from the bladder, hair loss, sterility, and, years later, some patients may even develop cancer from its use. When kidney failure occurs very rapidly in patients with lupus (acute renal failure), a series of extremely large doses of corticosteroids and/or Cytoxan given intravenously (pulse therapy) may be helpful.

Patients who do not respond to treatment may progress to kidney failure, requiring dialysis or a kidney transplant. Both dialysis and kidney transplant may result in excellent long-term improvement in the patient's condition. During hemodialysis (see Figure 3), the patient's blood is pumped past a special

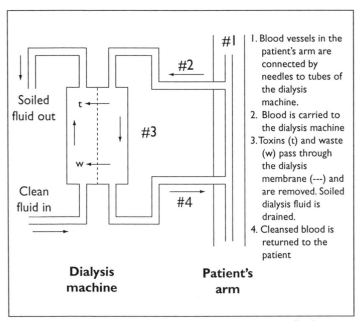

Figure 3. Diagram showing steps in hemodialysis

membrane on the other side of which is a special cleansing solution. Toxins and waste products which have accumulated in the blood pass through the membrane and the blood is cleansed. Usually this process is repeated three times each week. Each session lasts anywhere from 4 to 6 hours. Peritoneal dialysis is sometimes used instead of hemodialysis, especially when dialysis will only be needed temporarily. In peritoneal dialysis, the cleansing fluid is placed in the patient's abdominal cavity (the space that surrounds the internal organs: the stomach, the bowel, the liver, etc.) and the lining of this cavity serves as a natural dialyzing membrane. Patients who have kidney failure which is advanced enough to require dialysis develop a natural suppression of their immune system and this may arrest the lupus throughout the rest of their body. As a result, lupus dialysis patients do as well as other dialysis patients who do not have lupus.

There has also been great success with kidney transplants in lupus patients. Kidney transplantation works best when a patient's lupus is inactive at the time of the transplant. Kidneys for transplantation may come from either relatives or unrelated organ donors. In order to decrease the chance of rejection (the lupus patient's immune system attacking the transplanted kidney), the tissue type of the donated kidney should match the tissue type of the patient as closely as possible. Cyclosporine, and other newer related immunosuppressive drugs given to kidney transplant patients, have significantly improved the success rate of transplants. Once the new kidney has been accepted by the body, recurrence of lupus in the kidney is rare.

To sum up all of this, we can now say that kidney disease, once the most dreaded consequence of lupus, is now often very successfully treated!

CHAPTER 8. NEUROLOGIC COMPLICATIONS

Michael M. Margolin, MD

Systemic lupus erythematosus (SLE) frequently affects the nervous system. It is estimated that anywhere from one third to three quarters of patients with SLE will experience some nervous system effects.

Table 6. THE MORE COMMON SERIOUS NEUROLOGIC PROBLEMS CAUSED BY LUPUS*

PROBLEM	PERCENT HAVING IT
Impaired thinking/alertness	20%
Seizures	15%
Decreased sensation/strength in feet	10%
Mental illness	10%
Stroke	5%
Involuntary movements	3%
Spinal cord problems: paralysis, etc.	1%

* *The percentages are only rough estimates based on combining the results of several different studies.*

Rarely, the very first sign of lupus may be a problem with the nervous system. Then it may be a neurologist who makes the diagnosis of lupus. A large variety of different nervous system problems can occur in lupus. The most common of the more serious of these are listed in Table 6.

In order to appreciate how this variety of neurologic problems can come about, it helps to understand how important the nervous system is to the body and the wide variety of functions it performs. The nervous system includes the brain, spinal cord, and the peripheral nerves (nerves outside the brain and spinal cord). The brain coordinates information for all other parts of the nervous system and has centers for sight, speech, thinking, memory, and personality. The brain is attached to the spinal cord and the connecting portion at the base of the brain is called the brain stem. The brain stem contains nerve cells that control the muscles of eye movement, facial expression, speaking, and swallowing, and other cells which aid in hearing and balance. The spinal cord contains nerve cells and bundles of long nerves that send impulses to and from the muscles of the body and the limbs and that receive sensory information from the skin and joints. This includes information about position, pressure, touch, and pain.

There are several possible ways that lupus can damage the nervous system. First, the blood vessels of the brain may themselves be damaged leading to bleeding (hemorrhage) or poor blood flow and death of tissue in the brain or brain stem. The patient affected in this way is said to have suffered a stroke. Second, the immune system may produce antibodies that attack the nervous system.

Changes in thinking are quite common in lupus but usually very mild.

Some of these antibodies attack nerve cells directly (antineuronal antibodies and so-called antiribosomal P protein) and others (anticardiolipin antibodies) result in the formation of blood clots. Third, there may be inflammation of the blood vessels and other tissues.

When lupus affects the nervous system, the type of problem the patient experiences depends on what area of the nervous system is involved and, as a result, what sensory and motor pathways are damaged. When there is general involvement of the brain, a patient may demonstrate what is called organic brain syndrome. This condition involves a diminished ability to think and remember. Most often these changes are very mild and can only be detected for certain with special neuropsychological testing (discussed in Chapter 9). Patients with more serious organic brain syndrome feel less alert and become lethargic. In the most serious cases, they may even lose consciousness and fall into a coma. The treatment of this serious kind of brain involvement in lupus usually involves high doses of corticosteroids.

Another complication due to brain involvement is seizures (sometimes called convulsions or fits). The occurrence of seizures may not signal the presence of severe lupus and the seizures can often be controlled with anticonvulsant medication (Dilantin, etc.) used to treat people without lupus who suffer from epilepsy. Seizures occur most commonly in lupus patients with kidney disease. Controlling the chemical imbalance caused by poor kidney function also helps to control the seizures.

Damage to the peripheral nerves is the next most common neurologic problem which is encountered in SLE. This usually takes the form of numbness and abnormal sensations (so-called "pins and needles") and inability to feel temperature change, vibration, or change in position, as well as in weakness of the muscles in the legs and arms. These changes affect the feet and hands predominantly and doctors refer to this effect as having a "stocking-glove" distribution. If the changes are severe, patients may inadvertently burn or stick themselves by picking up a hot pan or stepping on a nail, etc. This kind of damage can lead to infection and patients with peripheral nerve problems should consult a physician immediately if an injury is detected and should inspect their feet carefully for sores and puncture wounds.

Personality changes and even mental illness can occur in lupus. Personality changes are usually mild. The person experiences slight depression, anxiety, irritability, or even an unnatural feeling of well-being (euphoria). Much less often actual mental illness develops. The mentally ill patient has difficulty separating what is real from the distorted ideas in his or her mind. Hallucinations (usually hearing things that are not there) or delusions (false beliefs) may be experienced. The mental problems in SLE often respond well to medications used to treat mental illness in general but corticosteroids are often added as well.

As mentioned before, lupus can also cause strokes in which there is the abrupt onset of neurologic symptoms. Strokes give rise to a variety of abnormalities, including loss of sensation on one side of the body, loss of movement (paralysis) on one side of the body, problems with speaking and understanding speech, or problems with vision. The exact symptoms depend on what blood vessels in the brain are affected. Strokes are most likely in SLE patients who have the lupus anticoagulant, anticardiolipin antibodies or the antiphospholipid syndrome and/or high blood pressure. To prevent strokes, patients are given medication to control blood pressure (antihypertensives) and in cases where the stroke is due to blood clots, they may be treated with blood thinning medication (coumadin, for example).

An uncommon complication of lupus consists of repeated involuntary movement, so-called "chorea". The movements are jerky and usually affect one leg or arm or one side on the face. The cause of these is not well understood. Chorea can sometimes be treated by medicines used to treat other abnormal movements. Spinal cord involvement (myelopathy) in SLE is very rare but can be disabling. Patients with myelopathy develop weakness in both legs (paraplegia) or even in both arms and legs (quadriplegia) depending upon what level of the spinal cord is affected. Sensations from the paralyzed limbs are also affected. Since the spinal cord is critical for the control of bowels and bladder, incontinence may be a problem. When myelopathy occurs early in the disease before the diagnosis of lupus has been made, other neurologic diseases, such as multiple sclerosis, may be suspected. In SLE, myelopathy often can be treated successfully with high doses of corticosteroids.

Not all weakness which occurs in SLE is due to direct damage to the brain, the nerves, or the spinal cord. Sometime the muscles themselves become inflamed (myositis). This condition primarily affects the muscles of the upper legs and the upper arms. (Its diagnosis and treatment are discussed in Chapter 2.)

Besides the most common nervous system problems in SLE discussed above, many others are recognized but very seldom encountered. These include increased pressure of the fluid inside the brain causing headaches and visual loss, inflammation of the lining of the brain (meningitis), and inflammation involving a single nerve (mononeuritis) which can cause weakness in one foot (foot drop) and one wrist (wrist drop). Visual problems can also result from brain involvement in lupus. (These are discussed further in Chapter 11, on the eye.)

Diagnosing the nervous system problems in lupus can be very challenging. That is primarily because patients with lupus are often on corticosteroid treatment. This treatment by itself can bring about mental changes, cause weakness, affect the pressure of the fluid in the brain and affect vision, disrupt the chemical balance within the body, cause high blood pressure, and increase the likelihood of infection. In turn, infection can cause fever as well as many other problems which mimic lupus. Finally, other medications used to treat SLE can cause nervous system abnormalities similar to those we've been discussing. (Nonsteroidal antiinflammatory drugs can cause meningitis and drowsiness; Plaquenil can cause muscle weakness and visual problems, etc.) When a patient with SLE develops a neurologic problem, special tests are often necessary to determine whether the problem is due to lupus (then corticosteroids might have to be increased or immunosuppressive medication added), infection (antibiotics might be needed) or a side effect of medication (a change or a decrease in medicine would be necessary). Helpful in this determination are magnetic resonance imaging (MRI scans), computerized axial tomography (CAT scans), analysis of fluid drawn from around the spinal cord (by a spinal tap), recording of electrical activity in nerves and muscles (nerve conduction study and electromyogram), a variety of blood tests and blood cultures, and neuropsychological testing. (The latter is discussed in Chapter 9.)

Chapter 9.   Neuropsychological Testing

Sandra Koffler, PhD

Patients diagnosed as or suspected of having, systemic lupus erythematosus (SLE) may be referred by their physicians for a special series of tests of brain function called a neuropsychological examination. There are many reasons that such an examination may be requested. Patients with lupus often complain of problems that suggest possible involvement of the central nervous system and, in particular, the brain. It has been estimated that some disturbance in brain function occurs in at least 50% of SLE patients. This disturbance (discussed in Chapter 8) may be expressed as headaches, memory problems, confusion, visual disturbances, seizures, or personality changes.

The onset of neuropsychological problems may be an early warning sign of lupus activity (in which case the person is said to have an "organic" problem) or it may be a reaction to the stress of having a serious chronic illness (in which case the person is said to be suffering a "functional" illness). Both the patient and the doctor often have difficulty telling the difference between a disorder which is caused by the disease as opposed to one which is caused by other problems in the patient's life. At the present time, there is no one sure laboratory test to detect lupus-related central nervous system involvement.

A second reason for the doctor's referral for testing may be to check for side effects of treatment, especially treatment with steroids. Psychological effects of steroids may range from very mild changes in mood to more disturbing mental illness. Neuropsychological testing may be helpful in providing clues to differentiate medication-induced conditions from problems due to lupus itself. If psychological effects are related to steroid therapy, they may be eliminated by simply lowering the dosage of the drug or, if possible, withdrawing the drug altogether and substituting some other form of treatment.

Some doctors refer all new SLE patients for neuropsychological testing.

Some doctors refer all recently diagnosed lupus patients for neuropsychological testing, including those who have no history or current evidence of a

---

Table 7. TESTS TO EVALUATE EACH SIDE OF THE BRAIN*

LEFT BRAIN FUNCTION	RIGHT BRAIN FUNCTION
Language and arithmetic skills	Perception of spatial relations
Recognition of language sounds	Recognition of rhythms and tones
Verbal memory	Visual memory

* In a right handed person. In left-handed people, the functions of each side are not always predictable. See the text.

---

central nervous system disorder, since these tests can detect mild or unsuspected brain disease. The purpose of this early testing is to obtain baseline information to aid in monitoring the course of the patient's illness and thus help to assess the effects of treatment.

Most people have encountered psychological testing in the form of intelligence testing or as part of an examination to see whether someone has an aptitude for a special type of work. What then is a neuropsychological evaluation? Neuropsychological testing examines specific behavior to determine the presence or absence of a problem in the brain. The "neuro" in "neuropsychological" means that the behavior which is being examined by the test reflects particular brain function. An example of such behavior might be drawing a copy of a sample figure. Such behavior is typically independent of how smart an individual is or what his or her personality is like. How a person goes about doing such a task provides more useful information than whether or not the figure is copied correctly. The neuropsychologist, the person giving the test, has special training and experience that qualifies him or her to look at abnormal results and suggest a possible cause of the disorder and possibilities for recovery. The neuropsychologist may also offer recommendations to help in the management of a patient's problem and may consult with patients and their families to help them understand the nature of the problems.

Neuropsychological tests can be classified into two broad categories: tests of general functions and tests of specific abilities. Although the boundaries are not rigid, tests of general functions examine complex behaviors such as memory, attention, reasoning, judgement and planning. Specific functions evaluated by neuropsychological tests include language skills (expression, comprehension, reading, writing), numerical abilities, motor performance, sensation and perception. Whereas the findings of the general tests may suggest the possibility of brain dysfunction, measures of specific abilities help to identify an area or areas of the brain that are associated with the problem. A first step is often to compare the abilities of the two sides (the hemispheres) of the brain, each of which serves quite different functions. Each side controls movement on the opposite side of the body. In a right-handed person, the left side of the brain governs speech and logical thinking (and is said to be "dominant"), while the right side of the brain is more concerned with artistic matters. In a small number of the left-handed, all language is in the right hemisphere and in many some language function may be represented on the right side. Table 7 lists types of tests used to evaluate each side of the brain.

Most often it is the cognitive or the more general neuropsychological functions that are affected in central nervous system lupus. Of the specific functions, complex visual perception, such as is required in mentally rotating an object to match a model, in finding subtle differences between two visual designs, or in tracing a path through a maze, tends to be affected.

In addition to tests of mental functions, tests of personality are included in the neuropsychological battery. They are included to see if there are psychological problems such as depression that are contributing to the patient's difficulties. If psychological problems are present, an effort is made to see whether they are actually a result of central nervous system lupus or associated with the individual's reaction to the illness.

The newest additions to the neuropsychological test battery are computer driven tests. These represent an important advance in diagnosing brain dysfunction. Because of the computer's ability to make accurate measurements of the test responses, to administer the tests in precisely the same way every time (no two human test givers would give the instructions in exactly the same way), and to keep track of a lot of details about the patient's history, mild problems or changes in a person's functioning can be detected and related to other facts about his or her condition. Other advantages are that computerized tests typically take less time to give than person-to-person tests, and, perhaps because of their resemblance to computer games, are often found by patients to be more interesting.

When all of the neuropsychological tests are completed, a final report is compiled. The report is based on the pattern of results on different tests **Test results are interpreted by comparison with standard results from similar healthy people.** and takes into account other important considerations. Such considerations include the patient's sex, age and level of education. The patient's results are always compared to standard test results gathered from healthy individuals of the same age and sex who have a similar background and education. The patient's medical and psychiatric history is also considered in the final report since some medication or an illness other than lupus could be contributing to abnormal test results.

The first reports of the effectiveness of neuropsychological testing in uncovering the presence of central nervous system lupus appeared in 1985. Since that time, this type of testing has proven to be a reliable and sensitive measure of brain involvement in lupus and a valuable addition to the usual medical examination and laboratory tests.

CHAPTER 10. PSYCHOLOGICAL EFFECTS

James L. Stinnet, MD

Patients with SLE often have psychological symptoms. These include such feelings as anxiety, sadness, depression, and confusion. Usually the symptoms are mild and don't interfere with normal daily functioning. Such symptoms are similar to those experienced by any patient with a chronic medical condition such as diabetes or heart disease. Sometimes these symptoms become more severe and cause patients real emotional distress by interfering in their daily activities or in their relationships with others. When this occurs it is important that patients discuss the problems with their doctors. The doctor can do some investigation to find out what may be causing the problem and can suggest appropriate treatment.

Various Causes Of Psychological Problems

Some people, unfamiliar with lupus, might look at a patient who is very upset emotionally and think, "Who wouldn't be upset if she (or he) had a serious illness like lupus? That's just a normal response." Although this

Any chronic illness affects mood and relations with others.

thinking has some truth to it, it doesn't do full justice to the complexity of the situation. Experts in the field of lupus and psychology generally divide the emotional problems experienced by patients with SLE into four categories: (1) responses to the stress of illness, (2) direct effects of lupus on the brain, (3) indirect effects of lupus on the brain, (4) side effects of medication.

Response to the Stress of Illness

Response to the stress of a chronic illness is the most common reason for the lupus patient to experience emotional distress. It is simply the direct result of experiencing the state of being ill. Illness is a complicated condition. It includes the physical sensations caused by the illness (for lupus these often include pain, a feverish feeling, and fatigue); changes in self-image due to changes in appearance (for example, skin rash, shallow complexion, weight gain, "moon" face from steroids); and changes in interpersonal relations. Other people may take over the sick person's responsibilities, exclude the sick person from certain activities, "baby" the sick person, etc. In other words, the person who is ill changes – physically, psychologically, and socially. Anger, sadness, fear, anxiety, guilt, shame, and frustration are normal, although undesirable, responses to being ill. Patients who experience these feelings should be reassured that they are not mentally ill.

Direct Effects on the Brain

As discussed in an earlier section on neurologic changes in lupus (Chapter 8), SLE has many direct effects on the brain. Typically these take the form of problems with memory, slowing of thinking, confusion, or hallucinations. They may, however, show up as anxiety or depression. Then neuropsychological testing (Chapter 9), special scans of the brain, and blood tests may be useful to sort out whether active lupus is playing a role in the mental and emotional problems.

Indirect Effects on the Brain

Just as in other chronic diseases, when lupus affects the kidneys, the lungs, the heart, or other organs, there may be indirect effects on the brain. Disease of the kidneys can cause high blood pressure, allow waste products to accumulate in the blood, and change the normal balance of chemicals in the body. Heart and lung disease can affect the amount of oxygen the brain receives and can also affect chemical balance. Thus, when people have lupus affecting these organs and also have psychological symptoms, it is important to try to treat that organ disease before attributing the psychological problems to other causes.

Side Effects of Medication

Many medications used to treat SLE, and its associated problems such as high blood pressure, have psychological effects. Most outstanding in this regard are corticosteroids. Psychological effects appear related to the steroid dose, higher doses causing more emotional problems than lower. Steroids often cause a kind of "high." The patient is more energetic, has a greater appetite, and becomes more elated and outgoing. Higher doses may cause insomnia, nervousness, and irritability. Emotions may become labile (mood switches rapidly; the patient laughs one minute and cries the next). Rarely corticosteroids cause even more pronounced effects with the development of hallucinations and confusion.

Not all people on steroids develop these side effects. Besides the size of the dose taken, side effects depend upon how rapidly the dose is changed as well as individual differences among people. For reasons that doctors do not yet understand, some people can take even high doses of steroids for a long time with little or no obvious emotional effect.

Besides corticosteroids, many other medications have been reported to have psychological effects on some people. Thus, when a patient reports this kind of problem to the doctor, one of the first things the doctor thinks about is whether the patient might be experiencing the side effect of some drug, particularly a drug that has recently been started or increased.

Types of Emotional Response

In the discussion above about different causes, we mentioned briefly various emotional problems which patients with SLE might have. In this section, we will discuss in more detail several of these problems that occur commonly. They can be grouped into categories we will call mood states, cognitive dysfunction and psychosis.

Mood States

All of us experience various mood states as a natural part of being human. Our moods are always in the background, coloring how we perceive the events in our lives. Some common moods are happiness, optimism, contentment, anger, fear, guilt, sadness, and anxiety. The two most common moods that trouble people with SLE are anxiety and sadness. As we noted before, these are natural moods for anyone with a serious chronic illness and are not to be taken as a sign of mental illness.

It is easy to understand why patients with lupus would suffer from anxiety. Many questions bother them for which they have no good answers. Will they get sicker and feel worse? Will they be able to afford medical care? Will they be able to meet their responsibilities at home or on the job? Will their family understand what is happening to them? Will they die? Because of these upsetting thoughts, it is often tempting for the anxious patient to seek relief through the use of medications known as "tranquillizers." Patients often request these from their physicians; and doctors, in an attempt to be helpful, commonly prescribe them. In fact, tranquillizers (Valium, Xanax, Librium, Equanil, etc.) are not appropriate in this setting. They are habit forming and can cause actual addiction. Moreover, they do not help the sadness that often accompanies the anxiety seen in chronic disease. The best treatment for anxiety is to talk about the feeling and get it out in the open. Often, discussion with a health care provider or meeting with a support group made up of others who have the same illness is all the treatment needed to allow a patient to deal appropriately with this kind of psychological problem. (Support groups are the subject of Chapter 19.)

Sometimes patients and doctors mistake sadness for depression and assume wrongly the sad person is mentally ill. Sadness is a reaction to sickness. It waxes and wanes along with the illness and other events in the patient's life. People who

Sadness is not the same as depression.

are sad can be distracted and experience other moods that replace sadness. Thus a woman with active lupus who is saddened by her disease may feel joyful at the sight of a new grandchild. People who are depressed, on the other hand, are always "down" even when the event that triggered the depression has passed or when something "good" has happened. A depressed woman with active lupus may feel terribly unhappy even when the flare of her disease has passed and she may be unable to delight in events such as the birth of a grandchild. In addition, depressed individuals often suffer from inability to sleep (sometimes awakening in the early morning hours), appetite problems (decreased or increased), loss of sexual drive, irritability, and loss of interest in activities they previously found engaging such as reading, visiting with friends, watching television, etc. Depression represents a mood change carried to the extreme of mental illness and requires special treatment. Sadness can usually be treated like anxiety, by talking about the problem with others who are knowledgeable and sympathetic. Depression requires more formal treatment. A variety of effective antidepressant medications are available. Severe depression calls for care by a psychiatrist and may require a brief period of hospitalization.

Cognitive Dysfunction

Cognitive dysfunction is confused thinking or

mental "clouding." It is often caused by physical illness and is part of what is called organic brain syndrome. In lupus, as described above, it can be due both to the direct and indirect effects of lupus on the brain. These confused thought processes can be expressed in several different ways. People may become disoriented; they may be unable to recognize time or place. They may even be unable to tell what they are doing or who they are. There may also be problems of attention span; people with cognitive dysfunction may be easily distracted and forget their place in a book or a conversation. Even simple calculation becomes difficult. Following a familiar route may be tricky, and memory, especially for recent events, is poor.

Treatment for cognitive dysfunction usually centers on treatment of the underlying physical cause, although patients may benefit to some extent from retraining or the use of devices to aid memory.

Psychosis

Very rarely, patients with SLE may suffer psychosis. Psychosis is severe mental illness that causes a break from reality. A person who is psychotic cannot tell the real world from an unreal world in his or her head. The psychotic suffers from delusions (believing things that are not true) and/or hallucinations (hearing or seeing things which no one else can hear or see). A common delusion is

Psychosis in lupus may be caused by high dose corticosteroids.

paranoid thinking. Those with paranoid thoughts often are convinced that someone or some group is plotting to kill them. They spend much of the time trying to protect themselves from imaginary enemies. They may believe doctors are trying to poison them with medicine or trick them into treatment. Hallucinations experienced by a psychotic usually involve hearing imaginary voices which suggest actions or make threats.

Psychosis in lupus is often a side-effect of high dose corticosteroids but can be a result of the effects of the disease itself on the brain. Treatment of psychotic symptoms always requires close cooperation between the medical doctor taking care of the lupus and a consulting psychiatrist. Psychosis usually can be treated successfully with antipsychotic medication along with changes in corticosteroid dose.

Summary

Emotional problems are common in SLE. Not all are due to the disease itself. Many are normal responses to illness. Most respond well to treatment.

CHAPTER 11. THE EYE

Stephen H. Sinclair and Ernesto L. Collazo, MD

Before we discuss eye problems in lupus, it will be helpful to explain the structure of the human eye. The parts of the eye may be compared to the parts of a camera.

The camera contains a lens that focuses an image onto the film located against the back wall of the camera. The eye is arranged in a similar fashion. It is protected by the eyelids which act as lens covers but

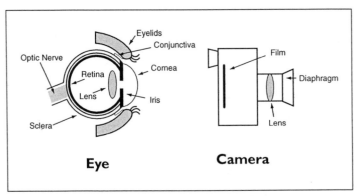

Figure 4. A diagram of the eye and a camera, for comparison

also perform like windshield wipers, blinking to spread tears over the surface of the eyes to keep them moist and clear. The lid has a smooth inner lining known as the conjunctiva. The conjunctiva is a membrane (something like a very thin skin) which also bends around to cover the front portion of the eyeball. It thus prevents objects such as dirt and contact lenses from getting behind the eye. The front surface of the eye is covered by the cornea, a transparent window similar to the crystal of a watch. Behind the cornea is the iris which may be of various colors (brown, blue, green, etc.). The iris acts similarly to the diaphragm of the camera by controlling the amount of light that enters the eye. Behind the iris is the lens which, like the lens of the camera, focuses the light. Instead of the film in the camera, it is the retina at the back of the eye which is the place where the image is recorded. The lens of the eye is not hard like glass but rather is a bag of clear protein. The outer wall of the eye, the sclera or the white of the eye, provides structural strength. The retina, the light sensitive layer that is similar to the film of the camera, lies flat against the back inside wall of the eye. The nerve impulses produced by images on the retina are transmitted to the visual part of the brain by the optic nerve in the back of the eye.

Eyelids

Lupus can produce inflammatory lesions (or sores) of the eyelids. The lesions may be small and individual ("discoid rash") or they may be more widespread. Sometimes they cause swelling, irritation and redness of he eyelids, and occasionally loss of the eyelashes. Over time, these lesions, if untreated, may result in scarring which can distort the eyelids and prevent blinking and proper cleaning of the front of the eye. Treatment is with corticosteroids taken by mouth or applied to the eyelids in the form of an ointment.

The Front Of The Eye

Rarely, the conjunctiva in lupus becomes inflamed causing redness and tearing. Since the tear glands are located there, inflammation of the conjunctiva may reduce tear production resulting in dryness of the eye. (This same inflammation may also affect the glands near the mouth which make saliva and those in the vagina which make vaginal secretions. The combination of dry eyes, dry mouth and dry vagina is one of the main features of a condition called Sjogren's syndrome that affects some lupus patients.) With reduced wetting, the cornea may lose its clarity, become roughened and irritated, and prone to infection. Very rarely, inflammation of the sclera or iris may also occur. Again, corticosteroids are used to reduce the inflammation. They are given by mouth or as eye drops. In addition, artificial tear preparations and ointments are used to reduce the dryness and subsequent irritation of the eye. Infection of the cornea, which may cause such symptoms as a foreign body sensation (the feeling that something has gotten into the eye), eye pain and blurred vision, requires prompt and careful treatment with antibiotics.

Lens And Cataracts

The clear lens capsule is filled with a protein gelatin-like substance. When a person has been focusing on a distant object and then switches to look at something up close, tiny muscles pull on the lens to change its shape, thus changing its focus. As we become older, the gel within the lens hardens and makes focusing more difficult. When we are young, we can focus on objects which are close up to our nose but, as the years pass, we must move things further away to focus on them. Older people find that their arms are too short to hold a printed page in a position where they can read it. This is especially true under conditions of dim light (standing at a public telephone under a street light, for example). In poor illumination, the iris has to open to enlarge the pupil and let in more light. This reduces the depth of focus and makes the job of the lens even harder.

A second problem that occurs with age concerns the protein gel of the lens. As we grow older, the gel of the lens tends to crystallize, creating glare or altering the focus. As this crystallization gets worse, the lens becomes cloudy and the glare or irregularities in focus reduce vision significantly. The cloudy lens is called a "cataract". People with SLE are especially likely to have problems with cataracts because one of the side effects of corticosteroids is to hasten these lens changes.

Cataracts may first come to attention because of increased glare, especially bothersome during night driving or in bright sunlight. In the early stages the glare can be reduced by wearing pale amber (yellow) tinted lenses for night driving or indoor reading, and dark amber (brown) tinted lenses to reduce the glare of the sun. Polarizing lenses can also reduce the glare. The focussing problems can be reduced by changing prescription glasses, although the results are only temporary since the lens of the eye continues to change. There has been much interest in anti-oxidant vitamins (vitamins E, C, beta carotene, etc.), herbs, and home remedies to try to prevent cataract formation, but so far carefully controlled studies have not shown these to have any beneficial results.

When changes in glasses and tinted lenses no longer provide reasonable vision, surgery on the eye, "cataract extraction", is required. The surgery is usually performed under local anesthesia (requiring an injection of anesthetic around and beside the eye) and does not require an overnight stay in the hospital. A small incision is made at the edge of the cornea and a hole is made in the capsule in front of the lens. Although we hear in the news media that lasers are used for cataract surgery, this is not really the case. A ultrasonic needle (one which transmits high energy sound) is put into the cloudy lens and the cloudy portion is liquefied. The liquid is then vacuumed out leaving the clear capsule behind and a small plastic lens is implanted into the capsule. The modern lens implant is very flexible and can be inserted in a folded position through a tiny incision that does not require any stitches. Once inside the capsule, it can be unfolded into the proper position.

Before the surgery, the lens implant which will provide the proper focusing power for that particular patient's eye is chosen.

Cataract surgery is extremely safe!

There is usually minimal discomfort after surgery and vision is very rapidly restored, often within days to weeks if the rest of the eye is working properly. Once the lens is inserted, however, its shape cannot be changed by the muscles of the eye. For that reason, the post-surgical patient will probably have to wear reading glasses or glasses for distance. Research is underway to develop a lens which can be focused, doing away with this need for glasses.

Cataract surgery is among the safest of the common surgical procedures. Rare complications are usually those associated with tearing of the capsule when the cloudy lens is removed. About 93% to 95% of all patients who undergo cataract surgery can look forward to seeing extremely well!

Retina

By far the most common effect of SLE on the eye involves injury to the blood vessels that supply the retina. Small retinal hemorrhages can result, as well as blockages of the smaller retinal blood vessels. These cause damage to the retinal tissue due to lack of an adequate blood supply. Infrequently, larger arteries may also be blocked leading to loss of function in large areas of the retina. When this involves the center of the retina, known as the macula, a large area of central vision is lost. The optic nerve itself may also suffer from blockages of the blood vessels which supply it, resulting in loss of vision in the entire eye.

In rare cases the blockages of blood vessels in the retina may be so severe and widespread that the body forms new retinal blood vessels. This process is termed "neovascularization." The new vessels grow out abnormally from the surface of the retina into the substance that fills the inside of the eye (the vitreous gel). The new vessels are prone to bleeding when stretched or pulled by the gel, resulting in severe vision loss. Although these abnormal blood vessels are rare in patients who are on adequate treatment for lupus, all lupus patients should be followed with periodic eye examinations because the blockages and abnormal vessel growth may occur without the patient noticing symptoms. If blockages or neovascularization are detected early, they may be treated with a laser. This procedure is usually done as an outpatient.

The Brain

When the brain is affected by lupus (see Chapter 8), the resulting damage may affect the visual system in a variety of ways. These include defects or gray areas of the visual field in one or both eyes, eye movement abnormalities which can lead to double vision, disturbances in the function of the pupils, and damage to the optic nerve leading to loss of vision in one eye. These problems can be difficult to diagnose and sometimes require consultation with a neuro-ophthalmologist, an eye doctor who specializes in eye problems connected with brain disease.

Drug Side-Effects

Treatment to control disease activity is vitally important to the well-being of the patient with lupus. It also helps to control the effects of lupus on the eye. Some

Antimalarials can affect vision. Safe use requires eye checks.

of the drugs which are used in the treatment of systemic lupus, however, can have side effects on the eyes. As we noted before, the long-term use of steroids may cause the formation of cataracts. In addition, corticosteroids can lead to the development of glaucoma, a condition in which an increase in the pressure within the eye causes damage to the optic nerve and an irreversible loss of vision. Glaucoma can be treated with medications to lower the pressure within the eye but early detection is critical for a good outcome.

Antimalarials are another group of drugs commonly used to treat SLE. One of the first of these to be used, chloroquine, was found to have a serious effect on the eye. It was found to accumulate over time in the layer between the retina and the sclera. This led, in some cases, to destruction of the central retina with resulting blindness in the middle of the visual field. A drug similar to chloroquine is more commonly used today. It is called hydroxychloroquine (Plaquenil). This drug appears to be less dangerous than chloroquine. At any rate, vision loss from antimalarials, in the relatively low doses currently used, is extremely rare. This is true even when the drugs are taken over several years. Lupus patients who are on antimalarials should have regular eye checks (at an average of every six months), however. They must be checked carefully for vision and visual fields, and evaluation of the retina. If damage to the retina is present, it can be detected early, and the drug can be stopped without any further injury to vision. Eye tests needed to check on antimalarial drugs are not entirely the same as routine eye tests. That's why it is essential that the ophthalmologist know when a patient is on an antimalarial drug or when it has been recommended that such a drug be started.

Eye Examinations

As we have pointed out in several of the sections above, many of the eye problems experienced by lupus patients can be corrected or controlled if discovered early. It is therefore important that every lupus patient have regular eye examinations. Because lupus is a serious medical disease with many possible complications involving the eye, it is recommended that these routine examinations be done by an ophthalmologist. An ophthalmologist is a physician (an M.D. or a D.O.) who specializes in the eye. He or she will recommend an examination schedule for each individual based upon such factors as age, the severity of the lupus, and the medications being taken.

Chapter 12. The Blood

Douglas B. Cines, MD

The blood contains three types of cells. These are the red blood cells which carry oxygen to the tissues, the white blood cells which play a major role in fighting off infection and regulating immune reactions, and the platelets which are important in the clotting of blood.

Red Blood Cells

When red blood cells are decreased, a person is said to have an anemia. Patients with mild anemia have no symptoms. As the red blood cell count falls, they feel fatigued because not enough red blood cells are available to carry oxygen to muscles and other tissues. Patients who are more seriously anemic may feel dizzy, experience a rapid heart beat or chest discomfort. These symptoms are more likely to develop during exercise when the body's demand for oxygen is increased. When a patient reports increasing fatigue or any of these other symptoms, the physician often checks to see if there is anemia present by ordering a blood count. The report of this count always includes the term "hematocrit". The hematocrit refers to the proportion of the whole blood occupied by the red blood cells. Usually about 40% of the blood is composed of red cells, but in patients with anemia, this proportion may be reduced to 20-30%

or less. If anemia is discovered, the physician can order other tests to find out the cause. In SLE, anemia comes about in four main ways.

Anemia of Chronic Disease

Normally, approximately 1% of red blood cells are removed from the circulating blood each day as a result of aging. The bone marrow, where all blood cells are made, replaces these cells with new ones. When lupus is active, many patients develop anemia because the bone marrow produces fewer red blood cells than are needed. The exact reason why fewer cells are produced is unknown, but in some

Not all anemia can be treated with iron pills.

way this is related to the inflammation caused by lupus. This anemia is known as the anemia of chronic disease and is also found in other conditions such as rheumatoid arthritis. In most SLE patients, this form of anemia is mild and produces no symptoms. It does not respond to changes in diet, vitamins, etc., but improves when the lupus is controlled.

Iron Deficiency Anemia

Iron is necessary to make hemoglobin, the protein in red blood cells that carries oxygen. Sometimes anemia in lupus is caused by iron deficiency. Iron deficiency is also a common cause of anemia in women who do not have lupus. It usually results from loss of iron over many years due to menstrual bleeding. Medications used to treat lupus, such as aspirin and other nonsteroidal anti-inflammatory medications, may cause irritation of the stomach lining leading to bleeding and resulting in iron deficiency. After the diagnosis of anemia is made the doctor can order tests to measure the amount of iron in the blood to determine whether the anemia is due to low levels of iron. Iron deficiency anemia is treated with iron pills but these have no benefit in other kinds of anemia. Severe, or rapidly developing, iron deficiency anemia may indicate that there is internal bleeding (as from a stomach ulcer) and further tests may need to be done to check on this possibility.

Anemia of Kidney Disease

People with SLE frequently develop kidney disease. The kidney makes a hormone called erythropoietin that is needed by the bone marrow to produce red blood cells. If the kidney is damaged and does not produce this hormone, the bone marrow will produce fewer red blood cells. The doctor will be able to tell by urine and blood tests if kidney damage is responsible for the anemia. If kidney function improves with treatment, the production of erythropoietin increases and the anemia improves. In recent years, it has become possible to make erythropoetin in the laboratory, which can then be given to treat the anemia of kidney disease. This exciting development has not only improved the anemia in kidney disease but is also of limited benefit in some other kinds of anemia.

Autoimmune Hemolytic Anemia

Anemia may also result from the production of an antibody that attaches to the red blood cells. This form of anemia, called autoimmune hemolytic anemia, occurs in approximately 5% of patients with lupus. Red cells coated with antibodies are quickly removed from the blood and destroyed by certain white blood cells, called macrophages, that normally destroy antibody coated viruses or bacteria as part of the body's defense against infection. If the production of new red cells cannot keep up with this destruction, the patient becomes anemic. The doctor can tell if red blood cells are being destroyed by looking at a blood sample under the microscope. In hemolytic anemia, there will be red cells whose shape has been altered and also a large number of newly produced red blood cells. The diagnosis of autoimmune hemolytic anemia is confirmed by a blood test known as the direct Coombs' test, which measures both the presence and type of antibody attached to the red cell.

The treatment of autoimmune hemolytic anemia depends upon its severity. If the anemia is mild, there may be no need for treatment. In one variety of uncommon autoimmune hemolytic anemia, called "cold-agglutinin disease", simple measures such as preventing exposure to cold temperature may be sufficient. For some patients, periodic transfusions of warmed blood are used to control symptoms. Patients with the more common, "warm-antibody" type of autoimmune hemolytic anemia may require various forms of treatment. Most commonly, corticosteroids are given by mouth to decrease the removal of the antibody-coated red blood cells by the macrophages. Those who do not respond to prednisone, or who require high doses to control the anemia, may be advised to have an operation to remove their spleen. The spleen is the organ of the body where most of the red cells to which antibodies have become attached are trapped and destroyed by macrophages. In some patients the hormone, Danazol, or other drugs such as cyclophosphamide (Cytoxan) may also be recommended. Transfusions are used only as a temporary measure since the transfused red cells will also quickly become coated with antibodies and will be destroyed.

White Blood Cells

The white blood cells include a number of different cell types many of which play a role in fighting infection. White cells, in general, are decreased in lupus and, partly as a result of this, patients with SLE may contract more infections than others do. There are typically no symptoms as a direct result of low white blood cells although when the total counts get very low, the patient may experience high fever as a result of infection. In this situation, in addition to antibiotics, it may be necessary to treat with corticosteroids as well as with a substance which stimulates white cell growth.

In SLE, the body attacks its own blood cells.

One type of white blood cell is especially closely

linked to lupus activity. That is the lymphocyte. Lymphocytes are divided mainly into two types, the B lymphocytes which make antibodies and the T lymphocytes which help to regulate the activity of the B lymphocytes and also help the body to recognize and attack foreign invaders. In lupus, the B lymphocytes are hyperactive, producing many types of antibodies, including many directed against the body's own cells (see Chapter 3). Some of the T lymphocytes, whose function it is to "help" the B lymphocytes, are abnormal, encouraging the inappropriate antibody production to go on. Certain of these antibodies are those which attack red blood cells, platelets, and the white blood cells themselves.

When a patient with active lupus develops a low white blood cell count, the doctor must always consider what medication the patient is taking. One of the most feared side-effects of the immunosuppressive drugs (Cytoxan, Imuran, etc.) is their tendency to depress the activity of the bone marrow and, as a result, the numbers of cells in the blood.

Platelets

Platelets are tiny pieces of cells which circulate in the blood. They come from bone marrow cells called megakaryocytes. Platelets release chemicals essential to the proper clotting of blood. Without enough platelets, a small injury to a blood vessel could cause severe hemorrhage. It is estimated that 25% of lupus patients have less than the normal number of platelets. This is due primarily to the fact that they produce antibodies against platelets. Fortunately, the number of platelets in lupus rarely gets so low as to cause bleeding. Because platelets rise and fall with lupus activity, in some patients the platelet count is sometimes used to help measure the activity of the disease. As is the case with white blood cells, low platelets counts may also be due to medications, especially the immunosuppressive drugs. Low platelet counts are also seen in the antiphospholipid syndrome (discussed in Chapter 2).

Dangerously low platelet counts can be treated with high dose corticosteroids and a number or other drugs as well as in surgical removal of the spleen.

CHAPTER 13. THE BONE

Marvin E. Steinberg, MD

Systemic lupus erythematosus (SLE) itself seldom has major effects on bone. As is the case with any chronic illness which decreases physical activity, it may cause a weakening of the bone. If there is inflammation around the joints, the bone next to the joints may be especially affected. In addition, since SLE is a disease which involves blood vessels, blood supply to the bone may be diminished or cut off entirely causing some bone to die. It is difficult in many cases to know how much lupus affects bone because most patients with significant lupus have to take corticosteroids at some time during their illness and these medications are known to have powerful effects on bone.

Corticosteroids such as prednisone are extremely effective agents for the treatment of certain aspects of lupus, but they do have certain side effects which can lead to complications in some patients. (For more on steroid complications see Chapter 5.) Two of the major complications involve the bone. The first is osteoporosis; the other is avascular necrosis. We will discuss both of these conditions in this chapter, reviewing the symptoms, the diagnosis, and the management.

Osteoporosis And Fractures

We can think of osteoporosis as a softening of

Table 8. SOME THINGS ASSOCIATED WITH OSTEOPOROSIS

Increasing age
Family history of osteoporosis
Female sex
Caucasian race
Decreased estrogen in females
Corticosteroid treatment
Decreased physical activity
Smoking
Alcohol
Decreased body weight
Poor nutrition
Kidney and liver disease

bone. If osteoporosis becomes severe enough, the bone is so badly weakened that it may break with only minor injury or slight increase in stress. Some degree of osteoporosis is a relatively normal condition which takes place as we get older, especially in the case of post-menopausal women. The prolonged use of corticosteroids accelerates this process. Table 8 lists these and some other important factors associated with osteoporosis.

Falls which injure the hip and the wrist are common and fractures or breaks in these bones are seen frequently in patients with osteoporosis. Breaks in the bones of the spine, known as compression fractures, can occur in osteoporotic people without any specific injury. They may result from a slight increase in the stress on the back such as occurs with bending, lifting, and even sneezing. Fractures of the wrist, hip, and many other bones of the arms and legs often need to be "set" or subjected to surgery. Compression fractures of the spine, however, usually need no specific treatment and heal by themselves. Rather than having a clean break through a bone with a separation between two broken parts, the bone of the different pieces which make up the spine, the vertebral bodies, crumble and simply collapse or compress in place. Often this happens so gradually that there is little or no pain associated and the patient is not aware that a fracture has occurred. A loss of height or a curvature of the back may be the only clues that compression has occurred. At other times the compression is associated with a sudden increase in stress on the spine and is very painful.

The only treatment necessary for these compression fractures of the spine is that which aims to relieve pain. Pain medications such as Tylenol, Darvocet or Percocet can be helpful. If the pain is severe, a few days to a few weeks of bed rest may be required, although doctors encourage patients to be as active as possible. A back brace or support is often prescribed which will help to support the spine, allowing the patient to get up and about without too much discomfort. Compression fractures of the spine usually become stable and the patient becomes free of pain somewhere between one to three months. At that time the back support is no longer needed and normal activities may be resumed. Then a good routine of back care should be started. This consists of exercises to strengthen the back and stomach muscles, and education designed to develop good habits for lifting and maintaining proper posture.

In recent years, an excellent test to diagnose osteoporosis has become **DEXA tests of bone are recommended for those on long-term steroids.** widely available. This is called DEXA, short for dual energy x-ray absorptiometry. A DEXA test is recommended for post-menopausal women and those people who have had to take corticosteroids long-term, as well as those with other risk factors for osteoporosis. Once it is recognized that a patient has osteoporosis, whether or not a fracture has already occurred, certain steps should be taken to prevent the osteoporosis from getting worse. The dose of corticosteroids should be kept as low as possible and the period of their use as short as possible. Weight-bearing exercise such as walking should be done regularly for at least 20 minutes three times a week to help preserve the strength of the bones. If patients are smokers or drink excessive alcohol, they are encouraged to stop. The diet should be well balanced with adequate protein, calcium, and vitamins (especially Vitamin D). Supplements are often prescribed to reach a total daily intake of 1000 to 1500 mg of calcium and 400 units of vitamin D daily. In post-menopausal women, estrogen is often added, providing there are no other health concerns to make this an unwise choice. Several drugs, some newly approved, are also often used to treat osteoporosis. One, calcitonin, previously available only in an injectable form, is now available as a nasal spray. Others, which belong to a different family of drugs called bisphosphonates are also widely used. One, etidronate (Didronel), is taken cyclically for two weeks out of every three months. The newest of the bisphosphonates to be approved is alendronate (Fosamax) which is taken daily.

The treatment of osteoporosis is not entirely satisfactory. Nothing works perfectly in all patients and the drugs are expensive and have side-effects which are sometimes poorly tolerated. The treatment program must be individualized for each patient and must continue over many years.

Avascular Necrosis

Avascular necrosis of bone is a disorder in which an avascular (lacking in blood supply) area of bone undergoes necrosis (dies). Avascular necrosis is not common, but is encountered in some patients with lupus. The area most often affected is the hip, in particular the upper part of the thigh bone (the femoral head) which makes up the ball of the ball-and-socket

---

Table 9. SOME THINGS ASSOCIATED WITH AVASCULAR NECROSIS

Trauma and fracture
Conditions causing blood clots
Blood vessel disease
Excessive alcohol
Corticosteroid treatment

---

hip joint. Other bones may also be affected, but much less often than the hip. These include the knee, the shoulder, and rarely the small bones of the wrist, foot or ankle.

In the general population, avascular necrosis of the hip tends to affect younger adults. In 50 to 60 percent of cases it occurs in both hips. The goal for treatment is to save the natural hip joint and avoid, if possible, having to remove the hip and replace it with an artificial joint. In order to accomplish this, early diagnosis is very important.

Many things can cause avascular necrosis. One of the most common is an injury or fracture of the hip which results in tearing of the blood vessels that nourish the femoral head. Avascular necrosis can also occur without major injury. Any condition leading to an abnormal increase in blood clotting such as antiphospholipid syndrome, a condition found in some lupus patients (see Chapter 2) can cause it. Avascular necrosis can also result from narrowing of the arteries seen in some blood vessel diseases. Although some authorities are of the opinion that the blood vessel changes of lupus itself (vasculitis) can result in avascular necrosis, there have been few, if any, cases reported in patients with lupus who have not been treated with steroids. Avascular necrosis also has occasionally been seen associated with excessive use of alcohol. A very small percentage of people who use corticosteroids for prolonged periods of time will also develop it. Why this is so is unclear. It may be that certain individuals are especially sensitive to steroids and form circulating fat droplets which block blood vessels as a result.

Within a few hours after the blood circulation to the bone is blocked, the cells in the bone begin to die. The body then makes an attempt to repair the damage. During this repair process the pressure within the bone begins to build. If only a small area of bone has lost its blood supply, this area often heals without treatment and the patient may not be aware that anything unusual has happened. If, however, the involved area is large, it will usually not heal and damage to the bone continues. The dead area of bone becomes weakened and begins to collapse. Eventually, the joint surface itself becomes involved, and actual flattening of the normally round femoral head results. The cartilage of the joint is subjected to abnormal stresses and undergoes gradual breakdown. Since this cartilage gets its nourishment from the fluid within the joint and not from the blood supply of the underlying bone, it remains alive for quite some time after the initial degeneration begins. In the later stages, cartilage damage ultimately leads to advanced degenerative arthritis (osteoarthritis) involving the entire hip joint. This series of events occurs in approximately 70 percent of hips in which a large area of bone has lost its circulation.

At first the patient with avascular necrosis has no symptoms. Later the build-up of pressure within the femoral head may cause a mild and vague type of pain. If the involved area is large, there is a steady increase in pain which may become quite severe. As the process continues, most patients develop a limp and note some decrease in motion of the hip joint.

Early on in avascular necrosis, x-rays are entirely normal. After weeks of symptoms, x-rays of the hip will show characteristic changes. An MRI (magnetic resonance imaging) scan is the best method for diagnosing early avascular necrosis. The MRI does not use x-rays but uses magnetic waves to show very early changes in the marrow of the bone, the bone itself, and other tissues in and around the hip joint. It is a very safe technique and is very accurate in diagnosing avascular necrosis.

In approximately 80 percent of established cases of avascular necrosis, the condition will progress if only "conservative treatment" is used. Conservative treatment consists of restricting activities and limiting the amount of weight the patient puts on the joint by having the patient use a cane or crutches. (The shoulder and knee do better with "conservative" management than the hip, and this is usually the treatment of choice for these joints).

Although there is no completely effective method for preventing avascular necrosis of the hip from progressing, there are a number of surgical procedures which are currently being tried and seem to show promise. These include drilling holes into the affected areas of bone to relieve the pressure, bone grafting, osteotomy (cutting a wedge out of the bone to change its position), and electrical stimulation to attempt to increase blood supply.

Once there has been definite flattening of the femoral head, these surgical procedures are seldom of much value. At this stage, patients should be treated conservatively with measures designed to decrease their pain and preserve function of the hip. These include restricting activities, prescribing gentle exercises, the use of a cane, and mild pain relievers. When pain and disability have progressed to the point that conservative methods of treatment are no longer effective in relieving symptoms, reconstructive surgery should be considered.

There are two commonly used procedures for reconstructing the hip: the replacement of only the "ball" of the hip with an "endoprosthesis" and the replacement of both the ball and the socket with a "total hip replacement". Of these two operations, the use of a total hip replacement seems to give the most consistent and durable results. Total hip replacement leads to

Total hip replacement is successful in the vast majority of cases.

complete or nearly complete relief of pain and relatively normal function in 90-95% of patients. Hips replaced nowadays should continue to function for at least 10 to 15 years in the majority of patients. In the younger individual they will rarely last a lifetime, but when they do wear out, the artificial hip can be replaced. Total hip replacement represents one of the most successful and one of the most popular surgical advances in the past 50 years!

Chapter 14. Teeth And Gums

Jay A. Denbo, DDS

Lupus patients may suffer from problems involving the teeth and gums due to the disease process itself. Some of these oral problems are indicators of disease activity. However, problems about the mouth also occur because of medications required to control lupus. COMMUNICATION, SELF-EXAMINATION, PREVENTION and KNOWLEDGE are concepts the lupus patient can use to minimize all of these difficulties.

Communication

Communication among patient, physician, and dentist is essential. Lupus patients should visit the dentist at regular intervals, usually at least every six months. Patients must keep their dentists informed about their medical histories and provide dentists with complete lists of medications with doses. Physicians should, in turn, be made aware of any dental problems and proposed dental treatment.

If the lupus patient needs dental surgery, communication between physician and dentist is especially important. In such cases it may be necessary for the dentist to consult with the physician to decide on the best management. To enable the patient to cope appropriately with the stress of surgery, a boost in steroid medication (or the reinstitution of steroids if the patient has been on them during the previous year) may be required. Nonsteroidal anti-inflammatory drugs may need to be stopped temporarily to prevent excessive bleeding. A prophylactic (preventive) antibiotic may be required if the patient has certain medical problems. Patients with damaged heart valves, those who have had artificial heart valves implanted, and those who have had joint replacement require prophylactic antibiotics before many dental procedures. Procedures which cause bleeding may result in mouth bacteria (germs) getting into the blood stream. Once in the blood they can travel to the heart valves and the artificial joint causing serious infection. The standard antibiotic currently recommended for prophylaxis by the American Heart Association is amoxicillin. A different antibiotic is substituted if the patient is allergic to penicillin (related to amoxicillin) or there are other unusual circumstances. Since healing may be somewhat prolonged and infection may occur more frequently in lupus patients, post-surgery follow-up examinations may have to be more frequent and extend over a longer period of time than would be the case for the non-lupus dental patient.

Self-Examination

Self-examination of the mouth should be performed regularly. Periodontal disease (disease of the tissue which surrounds and supports the teeth), which is a major cause of tooth loss in adults, usually does not cause pain and may not give any warning until significant tissue breakdown has occurred. However, there are clinical signs of periodontal disease which

Table 10. OBVIOUS SIGNS OF GINGIVITIS AND PERIODONTITIS

Bleeding gums
Red gum margins
Sensitive gums
Swollen gums
Loose teeth

the patient can detect with self-examination. Gingivitis (inflammation of the gum) involves infection by bacteria (germs) affecting the soft tissues (the gingiva, or gum) surrounding the teeth. Untreated gingivitis can spread into the tissues under the gum and become periodontitis. Periodontitis is a form of dental disease which is marked by thinning of the bone that supports the teeth and eventually leads to loosening and loss of teeth. Periodontitis is suspected when gingivitis is present. If any signs or symptoms of gingivitis or periodontitis are noted, the lupus patient should consult a dentist so that the problem can be accurately diagnosed and treated.

As seen in Table 10, there are several signs of gingivitis and periodontitis which the patient can easily observe. Gums which bleed for no reason or when eating or tooth brushing, and gums which are red, especially along the edges next to the teeth, are a sure sign of trouble. (Dark colored gums due to naturally occurring melanin, the substance which colors the gums in individuals with dark skin, is not an indication of inflammation.) Gums which are tender or painful on brushing as well as gums which are swollen with enlarged gingival margins (a condition in which a relatively thick edge of the gum is bound too loosely around each tooth) are abnormal. When gingivitis and periodontitis are far advanced, teeth loosen. At that stage, treatment by a dentist is the only treatment which is effective.

The self-examination should not be limited to the teeth and surrounding gingiva. A flashlight should be used to examine all of the tissues of the mouth. The floor of the mouth (the area under the tongue), the inside of the lips and cheeks, and the hard and soft palates (the top or ceiling of the mouth) should all be checked regularly for any red or white or irritated areas. If such areas are noticed, these should be brought to the attention of the physician and dentist. Approximately 25% of lupus patients have ulcers or other abnormal areas in the mouth. These are usually associated with a lupus skin rash (see Chapter 6). They can be found on the lips and on the tissue inside the cheeks. Ulcerations inside the mouth are areas which are red in color, feel sore and bleed easily. Such ulcerations may be indicators of disease activity elsewhere in the body and should be brought to the attention of the physician and dentist. Patients with oral ulcerations should not use denture powder or denture paste to retain removable dentures. If toothpaste irritates the mouth, baking soda and water or just water may be substituted.

Prevention

Prevention is the best treatment for cavities and for periodontal disease. Effective tooth brushing techniques will remove dental plaque which will prevent periodontal disease and tooth decay. Dental plaque is a thin film which is deposited on every tooth surface every day. Bacteria living inside the plaque cause gingivitis, periodontal disease, cavities and bad breath.

Gums that hurt or bleed should be brushed!

Most of the plaque accumulates between teeth and on the tooth surface next to the gum.

Putting toothpaste on a toothbrush and swishing the brush around the mouth for 20 to 30 seconds once or twice a day is not effective tooth brushing. Each tooth has five surfaces, the top or biting surface and four sides. The patient must clean all five surfaces of each tooth. The most critical areas are the parts of the tooth next to the gum; the junction between the gum and the tooth should be brushed very carefully. Soft bristle toothbrushes are recommended. The soft brush will remove plaque with the least irritation to the gum. It should take approximately 3 to 5 minutes to brush all of the teeth thoroughly.

The area between the teeth cannot be cleaned properly with a toothbrush. Dental floss, dental tape, rubber tips, pipe cleaners, special (interproximal) brushes to reach between teeth, stimulators and tooth picks are all useful to remove the dental plaque which accumulates between teeth. Any areas of gum sensitivity or bleeding or tooth sensitivity require effective plaque removal or the sensitivity and bleeding will get worse. A good rule is: If it hurts or if it bleeds, it must be brushed. Removing the plaque will reduce the bleeding and sensitivity. If the gum is unusually sensitive, soaking the toothbrush in hot water for a few minutes is recommended.

Patients who cannot use a regular toothbrush effectively, should discuss the various available electric toothbrushes with their dentist. Water irrigating devices which shoot water into the mouth do not remove dental plaque, can cut the gingival attachment to the tooth, and will increase the number of bacteria in the blood stream. For this reason, patients who are advised to take prophylactic antibiotics before dental procedures (see above) should also avoid the use of these water irrigating devices.

All removable dental devices such as full dentures, partial dentures and bite guards should be scrubbed with a stiff brush and soap at least two times per day. Germs of all kinds can be retained on removable appliances and can infect the soft tissues inside the mouth.

Knowledge About Specific Dental Conditions

Some lupus patients experience dry mouth (xerostomia). Dry mouth increases the risk of dental cavities and the risk of periodontal disease. Dry mouth can be controlled by chewing sugarless gum, sucking sugarless candies, taking frequent sips of liquid, using special mouth rinses as a saliva substitute, taking medications to increase the flow of saliva (sialogues), or using lubricants. Sipping liquid, chewing gum, or sucking candy is only effective for a short period of time and is not helpful during sleep. Sialogues and saliva substitutes require a prescription from a physician or dentist and can produce side effects which must be evaluated by the physician. Artificial saliva containing an ingredient called mucin is more effective than artificial saliva without mucin. Mucin containing lozenges are more effective than lozenges without mucin. Using no more than one-eighth of a teaspoon of a lubricant such as butter, margarine or vegetable oil to coat the soft tissues inside the mouth does not have any known adverse side effects and is temporarily helpful.

Facial pain affects some patients with lupus. It may originate in the muscles which control jaw movements or in the temporomandibular joint (TMJ) which is the jaw joint located in front of the ear. The pain can extend upward to the top of the head, forward into the cheeks, downward into the side of the neck, backward to an area just behind and below the ear and to the back of the head. Facial pain responds to over-the-counter analgesics (aspirin, acetaminophen, ibuprofen, etc.) mild muscle relaxant medications, heat applied to the painful area, ultrasound therapy, gentle jaw stretching exercises and bite-guard therapy (a plate worn between the upper and lower teeth at night to prevent grinding of the teeth). The most gentle and least expensive treatment is a jaw stretching exercise. In this exercise, the patient is required to consciously maintain a small space between upper and lower teeth during the day and to frequently open the mouth two or three inches, stretching the muscles used for chewing. This simple exercise, which can be repeated several times every hour, helps control pain originating from the muscles, keeps the muscles relaxed and decreases pressure on the TMJ.

Arthritic changes within the TMJ can result in a changing bite or a change in shape of the face. Separation of the upper and lower front teeth, which is referred to as a progressive anterior openbite, indicates bone changes within the TMJ. Patients who were able to bite thread with their front teeth find that they can no longer perform this task. This is a progressive condition and can not be corrected by dental therapy. A plastic bite guard can offer some relief to any discomfort associated with the openbite.

Some lupus patients, such as those with the antiphospholipid syndrome, are required to take coumadin, an anticoagulant medication. For such people, bleeding following dental surgery and tooth extraction may be excessive and these procedures should only be performed by a qualified specialist working in consultation with the physician and the general dentist. Dental examinations, cleaning and scaling, fillings and routine dental therapy do not cause significant bleeding and usually do not require any change in the use of anticoagulants.

Gingival enlargement (gum growing abnormally over the teeth) may occur in patients taking Dilantin, a medication used to control seizures. Keeping dental plaque from accumulating on the teeth will help to keep this enlargement under control. In extreme cases, surgery to remove gum may be required. Effective plaque control is essential to keep the gingival enlargement from recurring after surgical removal. Fungal infections can occur in the mouth. They are especially likely to form in lupus patients taking corticosteroids or immunosuppressive medication. The infection often appears in the form of a milky white patch that forms on the tongue or on the soft tissues lining the mouth. These white areas can be rubbed off leaving a sore, slightly red or ulcerated area, but to truly control the infection and prevent recurrence anti-fungal medications must be taken.

Summary

In the case of a patient with lupus, good dental care requires that the dentist work closely with the physician. Armed with COMMUNICATION, SELF-EXAMINATION, PREVENTION, and KNOWL-EDGE, the lupus patient can also become a member of the therapeutic team.

CHAPTER 15. CHILDHOOD DISEASE

Barbara E. Ostrov, MD and
Phyllis Slutsky, RN, MEd

About 20-25% of all lupus occurs in children. Lupus rarely develops under the age of 5 and only a small percentage of childhood lupus begins between the ages of 5-10. Childhood lupus most commonly has its onset during adolescence. Girls get lupus about three to seven times more often than boys before the age of 10, and about 9 times more often after puberty.

> **Childhood lupus commonly begins at adolescence.**

Family studies have shown that there are certain genetic factors called HLA types that are inherited and cause one child to be more likely than another to develop lupus. (See Chapter 4). Some children also inherit an inability to make certain immune system proteins (serum complement or antibodies) thus increasing the risk for developing lupus. When a susceptible person is exposed to a "trigger" such as a virus or other environmental factor, lupus may develop.

Systemic lupus erythematosus in childhood ranges from mild to severe and affects each individual differently. The usual course of lupus includes periods of "flares" (when symptoms are active) and remissions (when symptoms go away). Stressors such as infections (which occur more frequently in children than adults), and hormonal changes (which take place during puberty, menstruation, and pregnancy) may lead to lupus activity. In children, as in adults, sun exposure can bring on symptoms of lupus.

The initial symptoms of lupus in children can mimic many other conditions, and a thorough evaluation is necessary to make a diagnosis. Other conditions to be considered include juvenile rheumatoid arthritis, viral infections, Lyme disease, fibromyalgia syndrome, chronic fatigue syndrome, rheumatic fever and blood disorders.

Diagnosing lupus involves a detailed health and family history, a thorough physical examination and laboratory tests. Childhood lupus is identified according to the same guidelines developed by the American College of Rheumatology for the recognition of lupus in adults. (See Table 1, Chapter 1.)

The most common symptoms of lupus in children are rash, fever, and joint pain and swelling. Decreased appetite and weight loss are also common in children during the active phase of the disease. Inflammation of the kidneys (nephritis), inflammation of the covering of the heart (pericarditis), enlargement of the liver and spleen, and a low blood count may be more frequent in childhood lupus than in adult disease.

The rash of childhood lupus commonly affects the face but may appear on other areas of the body. Ulcers of the mouth and nose are common. Hair loss on the scalp may range from gradual thinning and change in texture to loss of large clumps of hair with resulting bald spots.

Central nervous system symptoms (affecting the brain and spinal column) are uncommon but may result in headaches, sei-zures, a change in memory or ability to think. Changes in the central nervous system

Fever, rash and joint pain are common first complaints.

can also affect vision, making it important to have eye checks by an ophthalmologist (a physician who specializes in diseases of the eye). A child's feelings of sadness or irritability do not necessarily mean there is central nervous system involvement. Changes in mood or behavior are common in children with lupus and may simply represent an understandable reaction to having an illness. If such changes are marked or otherwise worrisome, examination by a neurologist or a psychiatrist and diagnostic tests such as spinal taps, EEGs (brain wave tests), and CAT scans and MRIs of the brain can be helpful in deciding what changes are caused by lupus and which by the psychosocial stress of a chronic illness. (See Chapters 8,9, and 10 for related discussion.)

When the kidneys are affected by lupus, a urinalysis (examination of a small sample of urine) may reveal problems which can then be further investigated with a 24-hour urine collection and, in some cases, a kidney biopsy. Results of these tests are used as guidelines for treatment and the tests may need to be repeated for monitoring changes over time. (The kidney is the subject of Chapter 7.)

Lupus is most apt to involve serious complications when organs such as kidneys, heart or the central nervous system are involved. This involvement usually becomes obvious soon after lupus is diagnosed. As time goes on after the diagnosis of lupus has been made, the likelihood decreases that new body systems will become involved.

Extra care concerning sun exposure is important for all children with SLE. The use of sunscreens with an protection factor of at least "15" should be used on exposed areas of skin. A hat which shields sun from the face is also recommended. Planning the child's schedule to avoid sun exposure during the peak sunlight hours from 10:00 noon to 4:00 P.M. is recommended. Children themselves should be consulted when working out their schedules so that they understand the importance of any restrictions and will be more likely to abide by them.

Infections are common in childhood and children with lupus are especially susceptible. Families should be aware that fever and increased tiredness or shortness of breath may be a sign of either a flare of lupus or an infection and evaluation by a physician is often needed to tell which is occurring.

Children with lupus are entitled by law to an individual educational plan.

There are a variety of medications used to treat lupus. Many children are treated with a non-steroidal anti-inflammatory drug (NSAID) which helps reduce inflammation and joint pain. Aspirin, naproxen (Naprosyn), tolmetin (Tolectin), indomethacin (Indocin) and ibuprofen (Advil, Motrin, etc) have all been approved by the Food and Drug Administration (FDA) for use in children. Other anti-inflammatory medicines have not been FDA approved, but have been found to be safe in clinical studies of children. Anti-malarial drugs such as hydroxychloroquine (Plaquenil) are sometimes used to treat the rashes and arthritis of lupus. Because of possible eye toxicity, a child taking anti-malarials should be monitored by an ophthalmologist. Corticosteroids (prednisone, Medrol, etc.) are sometimes used to treat complicated lupus. The goal when using these medications is to use the lowest possible dose. As symptoms improve, gradually smaller and smaller doses are given with the hope that the medication can eventually be stopped altogether. When high doses of steroids are used over a long period of time before a child's full development is achieved, in addition to the side effects which are seen in adults, stunting of growth may occur. Giving steroids every other day instead of every day, helps to lower the chances of harmful side effects.

Some other drugs used mainly for kidney disease are cyclophosphamide (Cytoxan) and azathioprine (Imuran). These work to control the reaction of the immune system so that it causes fewer harmful effects on the body. Recent studies have shown that these drugs can be used safely in children and can control the more serious effects of lupus on internal organs.

A chronic illness like lupus has a very considerable effect on a child's life. During lupus flares, children often miss school. It is important that the family make contact with the school as soon as possible and stay in contact during the child's absence. A school counselor or nurse is often a good contact person. Depending upon how sick they are and how long they will be out of school, some children may need home or hospital tutoring while others may be able to do make-up work on their own. Because the course of lupus is so unpredictable, contacts with school authorities are often best made before a child gets sick so that tutoring can start right away if needed. Many rheumatology centers that treat lupus have a health care team that includes a social worker and a nurse who can help the family get the needed services.

Some children with lupus (like those with other chronic conditions) require an Individualized Education Plan (IEP). This includes an evaluation of all of the child's educational, psychosocial and physical needs which is done by a "study team" in each school district. The IEP identifies what each child needs in order to function well at school. Every child in the USA is entitled to this plan under federal law (PL#94-142). Chronically ill children are also entitled to vocational planning services in order to prepare for school or job training for their future employment. Each state has an Office of Vocational Rehabilitation (OVR) which offers career counseling that takes into account a child's physical abilities.

Any illness in a family member is likely to cause reactions in other members of the family. There is an increased burden on the family when caring for a chronically ill child. There may be added financial problems due to medical expenses and lost work time for parents.

Studies have been done to measure the effects on a family of a child's chronic illness. The families that coped best were those that did not cast their children in sick roles and so did not place undue limits on their daily activities. Families based on a solid marriage or with good support from larger family groups, friends or religious groups coped best with a chronic illness. Formal support groups for parents of children with lupus exist through the AJAO (American Juvenile Arthritis Organization) which is a part of the Arthritis Foundation. Support groups are an ideal way for teens to get the peer support and acceptance they need. Teens who attend these groups report a decrease in feelings of isolation and are better able to accept their illness. Because of the many issues and adjustments necessary for a teenager with lupus, however, individual counseling may be necessary for some.

A major problem for teenagers is coping with distressing changes in appearance which may be caused by lupus. These include rash and hair loss, often accompanied by acne and swollen cheeks due to steroids, and cause the child to question anxiously, "How do I look to the world?". Delays in normal puberty and sexual development may also cause young people with lupus to feel different than their peers. The onset of a female patient's first menstrual cycle may be at an older age than otherwise expected and the menstrual cycle itself may become irregular when lupus flares. It is important to discuss these possibilities frankly with the teenager, as the issues involved are often a major source of stress and worry.

Concerns about sexuality and pregnancy are often uppermost in the mind of the teenage lupus patient. Once sexual maturity is achieved, having lupus does not affect the young women's ability to become pregnant. Standard oral contraceptives which contain the hormone estrogen may cause an increase in symptoms of lupus and therefore are not typically prescribed when birth control is required. The hormone progesterone, used by itself, does not increase lupus symptoms and is an effective birth control agent. Progesterone is available as the mini-pill (taken like a regular birth control pill), an injectable drug given every 3 months, or a device that is surgically placed just under the skin and is effective for five years. Diaphragms and condoms are recommended as less effective alternatives for contraception (condoms, of course, should be used to prevent sexually transmitted disease). (More on this topic can be found in Chapter 17.)

It is highly recommended that a woman not become pregnant during an active period of lupus. Miscarriages (there is more "fetal loss" for women with lupus than in healthy women) or difficult pregnancies are more common when the disease is active. It is very possible to become pregnant and have a healthy baby, but careful planning with the doctor concerning the best time to begin, and what special precautions may have to be taken, is advised. There are many obstetricians available who specialize in "high risk" pregnancies. (Pregnancy is more fully discussed in Chapter 18.)

A unique type of lupus sometimes develops in the

infants of mothers who have lupus. This is called "neonatal lupus". It is associated with certain antibodies in the mother, especially those known as anti-Ro, though it develops in only about 25% of women with these antibodies. Neonatal lupus occurs more commonly in female infants. Infants with this type of lupus

Neonatal lupus may affect newborns of mothers with lupus.

typically develop a rash which is sun-sensitive and may have enlarged livers or spleens and abnormal numbers of some blood cells. Some of these infants may also be born with heart problems, including an abnormal, slow heart rhythm (congenital heart block). During the first six months to one year of life, the rash and the other problems disappear, but the heart problems may be permanent and require the placement of a pacemaker.

There has been a remarkable improvement in the prognosis of all types of childhood lupus during the past thirty years due to advances in diagnosis and treatment. Nevertheless, families of children with lupus need not only to seek expert medical treatment but to cultivate the support of their health care team, their school and their community.

CHAPTER 16. REHABILITATION

Bertram Greenspun, DO

Body systems affected by lupus that most commonly lead to the need for rehabilitation are the musculoskeletal system, the nervous system and the vascular system. Musculoskeletal system involvement may include muscle weakness and pain, tendon and ligament laxity and rupture, and arthritis. The joints may be swollen and painful and range of motion may be restricted. The central nervous system includes the brain and spinal cord. If the brain is involved with a stroke, there may be one-sided weakness, difficulty with thinking or memory, and trouble with speech. With problems in the spinal cord, paralysis or paresis (weakness) and absent or decreased sensation may occur, along with possible loss of control of the bowels and bladder. Various peripheral nerves (nerves outside the spinal cord and brain) may be affected with weakness and disturbed sensation in the arms or legs. Vascular damage done by lupus can cause decreased circulation to different parts of the body, especially the brain or the legs.

A physiatrist is a physician who leads the rehabilitaion team.

The PT helps to restore movement.

Some members of the rehabilitation team who can help the individual cope with these physical problems include the physiatrist, the physical therapist (PT), the occupational therapist (OT), the speech pathologist, the social worker, the vocational counselor, the recreational therapist and

> **The OT helps to re-establish the patient's activities of daily living.**

the psychologist. The physiatrist (pronounced fizz-eye-a-tryst) is a physician who specializes in physical medicine and rehabilitation and is the rehabilitation team leader.

The role of the PT is primarily to help the patient to be able to move around. This includes such everyday movements as getting in and out of a bed, on and off a chair, in and out of a car, and walking and climbing stairs. The PT can be especially helpful when joints don't move adequately or are unstable, when muscles are weak, when endurance is poor, when a loss of balance must be compensated for, and when pain limits activity.

The OT concentrates on restoring function with regard to activities of daily living. These include feeding oneself, dressing, going to the toilet, grooming, showering, and homemaking.

The speech pathologist can help with language problems such as slurred speech, inability to understand the spoken word or difficulty in speaking appropriately. The speech therapist can also be of benefit to those persons having trouble with swallowing.

The social worker is usually the coordinator of the assistance the patient needs from agencies outside the hospital or the doctor's office. The social worker arranges for equipment and services to be provided at home and is knowledgeable concerning resources available in the community for those who are ill or disabled.

The vocational rehabilitation counselor is typically a state employee whose job it is to arrange for retraining those patients too disabled to resume their previous vocations. Each of the states has an agency that provides vocational services to its residents. The name of such agencies varies from state to state but usually includes the word "vocational" or "rehabilitation".

The function of the recreational therapist is to involve the patient in some enjoyable leisure time activity that has therapeutic value. An example is the patient who is having a problem with weak or painful hands but is able to do a light activity such as painting a picture. This involves hand-eye coordination, choosing colors, and at the same time gives the patient an opportunity to socialize with other patients doing similar activities.

The psychologist is part of the rehabilitation team because every serious chronic illness brings with it psychological problems. In the case of lupus, the psychologist

Every effort is made to prevent a joint from stiffening.

helps to differentiate those sorts of mental problems from the kind unique to the disease itself and those due to medications used to treat the disease. He or she provides psychotherapy where it is indicated and aids in the decision to consult psychiatry when serious mental illness is suspected. (For more about this and related issues, see Chapters 8, 9 and 10.)

Exercise in various forms is a very important part of both physical and occupational therapy. When a patient is unable to move part of the body, passive range of motion is employed. The affected part is moved by the therapist to maintain healthy tissue and prevent contractures (joints that can no longer be moved through their normal range of motion). If the patient can move the body part to some degree the therapists will use active assisted range of motion. The therapist assists, but the patient does what he or she can to move the affected part. In almost every case some degree of strength returns. Muscle strengthening exercises can be added when appropriate. It is vital not to let any joint stiffen. If that happens, even though the muscles becomes active eventually, the joint may be so stiff and bent that it cannot be straightened out by the patient or the therapist. Preventing this problem is much easier than treating it.

It is important that the patient not overdo exercise since it is possible to make matters worse by overexertion. A good rule of thumb is that, if the individual remains overly fatigued or has increased discomfort for more than an hour and a half after exercise, the session was too strenuous and the next session should be made shorter or less strenuous.

If a joint is inflamed or sore, the muscles about that joint can still be strengthened by doing isometric exercises (tensing the muscles without moving the joint). Moving the joint may increase the pain when inflammation is present. Isometric exercises should be done without holding the breath as that tends to raise blood pressure. Family and friends can be instructed to help with exercise when appropriate.

Isometric exercise tenses the muscle without moving the joint.

Spasticity (very tight muscle with increased muscle tone), such as that which might occur with a stroke, can be treated with range of motion exercises. At times, ice massage will reduce spasticity; at other times, heat will work better. Application of heat or ice can be used on a trial and error basis since we know of no way to predict which will be more helpful for any individual. Either can be used easily and inexpensively in the home setting.

Sometimes the patient with lupus suffers from a localized area of diminished sensation. This may occur following a stroke or when there is damage to peripheral nerves in the legs or arms. Then something called sensory reeducation may be beneficial. This involves stimulating the insensitive area with different textures with the goal of reeducating the patient to the feel of that particular texture. The OT is usually the professional concerned with this process.

At some point, many people with lupus will have joint pain or stiffness. Joint swelling occasionally occurs but real joint deformities rarely result from the arthritis of lupus. An early morning shower can be quite useful in getting stiff and painful joints off to a reasonable start for the day. A hydrocollator pack is an inexpensive device that may help reduce joint pain and stiffness. This is a canvas bag filled with sand that can be heated in boiling water. When removed from the water and covered with several layers of toweling, it is placed on the involved joint for 15 to 20 minutes. This is best done before attempting range of motion exercises. It helps relax the tissues around the involved joint and makes the range of motion exercises easier. Ultrasound (the local application of very high frequency sound waves) is a way of giving deep heat and is the only means the PT has of getting heat into the area of a deep joint such as the hip. When used to improve joint motion, the range of motion exercise should be done at the same time the ultrasound is being used. The joint temperature will be the highest at that time and the tissues surrounding the joint will be the easiest to move. Ultrasound should be avoided when acute inflammation is present, when the joint itself is warm, or when it is red or tender to the touch as it can make the inflammation worse. Ultrasound is used primarily for joint problems which have persisted for days or weeks. For pain around joints which is only hours or a day or two old and for pain accompanied by signs of inflammation, ice is usually preferred over ultrasound or any other method of heat application.

MISTAKE: Putting a pillow under a painful knee!

Occasionally, when acute inflammation is present in a joint, it is best not to move the joint at all for fear of worsening the inflammation and causing more discomfort. Sometimes, in such a situation, the patient rests in bed. Then proper positioning is important to avoid muscle contractures and joints which don't move properly. The most common mistake made by patients is to put a pillow under a painful knee. If that practice is continued for a long

Thirty minutes of walking 3 times a week can be beneficial.

time, both the knee and hip on that leg may become bent and be unable to be straightened. Try walking with one hip and knee bent and you will understand why pillows under the knee should be avoided.

Exercise is recommended for everyone, including the person with lupus, in order to maintain cardiovascular fitness and to practice proper joint mechanics. If a pool is available, excellent exercise is possible without increasing pressure on painful joints. The warm water has a soothing effect and its buoyancy "unloads" the joints in the water. Walking is probably the best exercise for the individual with lupus whose legs are in reasonable condition. Since walking is a "weight-bearing" exercise, it can strengthen bone in addition to having good effects on the heart and the muscles. Thirty minutes of sustained walking three times a week will help increase cardiovascular fitness and prevent osteoporosis without resulting in joint damage. A reasonable schedule for the novice in poor condition is to undertake a five minute walk at a comfortable speed and increase the time walked by one minute every third day until the thirty minute goal is reached. Walking has to be sustained over a prolonged period to be beneficial.

Speaking of osteoporosis (more fully discussed in Chapter 13), there has been recent interest in the use of an especially designed backpack which can be worn while the person with osteoporosis is sitting upright or walking. It is reported to have beneficial effects on the bones of the spine which are prone to compress and cause a curvature of the back.

Because the person with either joint or central nervous system involvement may have problems carrying out activities of daily living, the services of an OT can be helpful. The OT will educate the patient concerning techniques of joint conservation (protecting the joint from damage) and energy conservation (completing a task while expending the least possible energy) which can be employed during routine activities. The OT will also makes splints to protect involved joints of the hands and arms. If movement has become a problem, the therapist can work on transfer techniques needed to allow the patient to get in and out of bed or on and off a toilet. Some adaptive equipment may be helpful. Something as simple as a raised toilet seat may make a great difference in a person's ability to manage going to the toilet independently.

Physical therapy helps before, as well as after, joint replacement.

There have been great strides in the last thirty years in the ability of the orthopedic surgeon to replace joints that have become devastated by disease. The joints most commonly replaced are the hip and knee. Therapists often are involved with patients both before and after joint replacement surgery. Prior to surgery, the patient is instructed as to what is to be expected during convalescence. For example, the patient scheduled for hip or knee replacement may be introduced to the use of a walker or crutches during the preoperative period. Since these devices rely on the use of the upper limbs, it is often useful to begin muscle strengthening exercises of the shoulders, arms and hands before surgery. After hip replacement, there are certain positions that should be avoided to avoid dislocation of the prosthesis (the artificial hip). It is best if patient education concerning this takes place before surgery. In the case of knee replacement, it is essential that range of motion be vigorously done following the operation and it is best to introduce the patient to these exercises before the prosthesis is in place. Many orthopedic surgeons order a CPM (continuous passive motion) machine immediately after surgery to assist with range of motion of the knee. This machine continuously, gently bends and unbends the artificial knee while the patient is lying in bed. The use of the CPM apparatus does not, however, substitute for the patient's own range of motion exercises.

Rarely, as a result of vasculitis or a problem with clotting of blood (antiphospholipid syndrome, etc.), the patient with lupus has to have part of a leg amputated. In most cases this will be a below-the-knee amputation. The physiatrist supervises the fitting of an artificial leg and the PT trains the patient how to put it on and how to use it properly to walk. The artificial limb is much lighter in weight and easier to learn to use in the case of a below-knee amputee than it is for an above-knee amputee. The below-knee amputee can usually be trained as an outpatient. The above-knee amputee usually needs inpatient training, especially if there are other areas of the body involved with lupus.

If, as in the case of the above-knee amputee, the person with lupus needs more intensive and complex therapy than can be provided as an outpatient, inpatient rehabilitation treatment in a special rehabilitation hospital or on a special rehabilitation unit of a general hospital is available. This may take the form of a regular admission with overnight periods spent in the hospital or it may mean admission to a so-called "day hospital" in which the patient spends most of the day, returning home at night to sleep. In any case, the inpatient care rendered in a rehabilitation setting is different from that given in the general hospital. On a rehabilitative unit, patients are expected to do as much as possible for themselves. That typically means that

Rehabilitation hospitals differ greatly from general hospitals.

they are out of bed as much as possible, and that they dress in street clothes and eat in a dining area, just as is done in the "real world". The rehabilitative team assesses the abilities of the patient on admission and, with the patient's active participation, establishes appropriate goals for the hospitalization. Weekly reviews are held by the team to assess the patient's progress and there may be one or more "family meetings" in which the "team" meets with the patient and the family/support people to anticipate questions and issues that may arise at the time of discharge.

In summary, there are many ways in which members of the rehabilitative team can help the patient with lupus. The special care they offer supplements the care given by medical doctors and surgeons, and often supplies that extra element which allows the patient with lupus to function normally. Lupus patients need to be aware of the potential value of rehabilitation so they can aid in their doctor's decision to request help from the various types of experts who make up the field of physical medicine and rehabilitation.

CHAPTER 17. SEXUAL RELATIONS

Mary Brassell, MA, CRRN

When one partner has a chronic disease such as lupus, many couples experience some type of sexual difficulty. Sexuality may be affected by disease symptoms, medications, or associated psychological factors. Physical changes brought on by lupus which may influence sexual activity include: oral ulcers, vaginal ulcers, arthritis, Sjogren's syndrome, and Raynaud's phenomenon.

Oral ulcers occur in about 10-15% of people with lupus. They can interfere with pleasant oral sensations. A prescription mouthwash with antibiotics or steroids may be necessary and can help heal the ulcers. Vaginal ulcers are present in less than 5% of women with lupus. They are rarely painful but when they are they can interfere with intercourse. A prescribed steroid cream or other medication can be used to treat them. Alternate forms of sexual expression (see below) can also be used until healing has taken place.

The vaginal dryness associated with Sjogren's syndrome responds well to the use of a water soluble lubricant which is absorbed and does not have to be removed. Water soluble lubricants (e.g. K-Y jelly) are available over the counter at drugstores or supermarkets. Vaseline-like ointments should be avoided since they can encourage infection.

The joint pain or arthritis that often accompanies

lupus may respond to warm baths, warming up exercises, and anti-inflammatory medication taken about an hour before sexual activity.

People with Raynaud's phenomenon have a condition in which blood vessels become narrower when they are exposed to cold. It can be very painful. Raynaud's can cause fingers and toes to change color and become very painful. To avoid this, some suggestions are: Avoid having sex in an air conditioned room. Wear socks if feet are sensitive to cold. Try a warm bath (not hot) prior to sexual activity to help open the blood vessels. During sex, blood pools in the genital area and less blood goes to the fingers and toes. Take the bottom position – it helps avoid the pressure on hands and feet that can further reduce blood flow.

Some medications influence sex life. Tranquilizers (anti-anxiety agents), anti-hypertensives (drugs that lower high blood pressure) and corticosteroids (prednisone, Medrol, etc.)) can affect both libido (sexual desire) and performance. Some anti-hypertensives decrease libido in men and women and produce temporary impotence in men (the inability to obtain or sustain an erection). Some people experience changes in libido while taking steroids. It is best to discuss such problems with your doctor, who may be able to make a change in your drugs so they won't interfere with sexual performance.

If a person with lupus develops low self esteem, unhappiness about the way her/his body looks, feelings of worthlessness, depression, fatigue, and feelings of inadequacy, the sexual relationship will certainly be affected. The patient may withdraw from his or her partner. The healthy partner may feel that this withdrawal means rejection and the loss of affection and love. If honest, open communication does not occur, the relationship may be in serious trouble.

Some medications given for lupus can influence sexual desire.

Sexual pleasure may be an important aspect of good health. Some studies have reported that arthritis patients are free from joint pain for up to six hours after intercourse. In that case, the sex act itself seems to be therapeutic. Even if intercourse is not possible, other forms of sexual expression such as cuddling, holding, stroking, kissing, and oral stimulation are all manifestations of sexual affection that can help reinforce a sense of self-worth and desirability.

Many publications contain various suggestions for different methods of sexual expression. The Arthritis Foundation has a publication titled "Living and Loving with Arthritis". It costs less than a dollar and can be obtained from the local branch of the Foundation. This booklet contains information about sexual expression, illustrations of comfortable positions to assume during sexual activity, and some sound advice about coping

Sexual pleasure appears to contribute to good health.

with sexual challenges. Suggestions for improving a sexual relationship are offered.

Sexuality is best thought of as another form of

communication that helps couples enjoy each other and deepens their intimacy in a loving relationship. Whether sexual problems are physical or emotional or both, willingness by both partners to discuss and search for solutions to sexual problems is essential. Help in reaching solutions may be obtained from physicians, from nurses in the field of arthritis and lupus, from psychologists, from sex therapists and from books available in stores and libraries. Information is readily available at low cost.

Family Planning

When the prospective mother has lupus, deciding to have a baby should begin with consultation between the prospective parents and the obstetrician, and should also include the rheumatologist or the primary internist. Several things need to be carefully evaluated. For example, is the lupus under good control or are there signs of an approaching flare? What medications are being taken? Do these medications have the

Deciding to have a baby deserves careful planning.

potential to harm the fetus (the baby as it develops in the womb)? If so, are these particular medications really needed to control the lupus or can they be omitted or changed? Are both prospective parents informed about possible risks to the mother-to-be or to the fetus as a result of lupus? (See Chapter 18 on Pregnancy) All of these issues should be investigated prior to conception and delivery. While women with lupus can have normal deliveries and healthy babies, those whose disease is not in good control have a greater risk of complications compared to those whose disease is well controlled. Some drugs used to treat lupus or its symptoms may prevent pregnancy or be harmful to the developing fetus. For example, cyclophosphamide (Cytoxan) sometimes causes sterility (inability to conceive a child) in the male or female and may cause abnormalities in the fetus. Prostaglandin E (misoprostol or Cytotec), sometimes given to protect the stomach when one is on steroids or non-steroidal antiinflammatory drugs, can bring about miscarriage. (When given along with methotrexate, it is even an effective way of producing a medical abortion.) If these medications are considered to be necessary for a patient with lupus, attempts at pregnancy should be postponed. Even after they are discontinued, the effects of certain medications may last several months, and pregnancy may have to be delayed.

If pregnancy is to be avoided, some method of birth control is needed. Avoiding sexual intercourse is, of course, a 100% foolproof method of birth control, but may not be either realistic or acceptable. Coitus interruptus (withdrawal of the penis from the vagina just before climax and discharge of the sperm) is difficult to achieve and apt to be very unsatisfactory. A condom worn to prevent venereal infection (AIDS, syphilis, gonorrhea) provides some measure of protection. A much more effective and practical approach to birth control is to plan for and use a specific method of contraception. Some contraceptive methods are not recommended for certain women with lupus. Other methods, which are medically appropriate, may not be acceptable because of religious beliefs. Still others may not be very effective, and an unplanned pregnancy, occurring when the patient is on dangerous medication or when lupus is very active, may result.

Contraceptive Methods

Contraception is a term that can be applied to many different types of birth control. Some block ovulation (the release of the ripe egg from the ovary), some prevent the egg and sperm from joining in the tube leading to the uterus, and some change the uterus lining so the fertilized egg (the egg **Many different types of contraception exist.** which has been joined by the sperm) is unable to attach and develop.

Different types of contraceptive measures include: barrier contraceptives (those which prevent the sperm from reaching the egg), spermicides (those which kill sperm), birth control pills or Norplant implants (female hormones which affect the reproductive system), IUDs (intrauterine devices which modify the inside of the uterus), fertility awareness methods (methods by which the couple can recognize when the woman enters a phase when it is "unsafe" – when intercourse may lead to pregnancy), and the "morning after" pill which affects the attachment of the fertilized egg to the uterus.

Barrier contraceptives include condoms, diaphragms, and cervical caps. If a condom is not applied correctly, or is removed too rapidly, there is a danger that some sperm may enter the cervix. If the diaphragm or cervical cap is not fitted over the entire cervix, sperm may be able to enter the uterus. Women using barrier methods must be instructed to make certain the appliance is applied fully over the cervix. (Masters and Johnson, as part of their famous sex studies, found that diaphragms were sometimes applied incorrectly, leaving part of the cervix unprotected). Learning how to insert a diaphragm requires know-how and practice if it is to be effective. Barrier methods can be made more effective by the addition of a spermicide. Spermicides in the form of creams, jellies, foams, sponges, and vaginal suppositories produce a film that kills sperm when they enter the vagina. Normal body temperature melts the spermicide causing it to spread around the vagina and cover the opening of the cervix. While some spermicides are supposed to be used with a diaphragm or condom, instructions for other types do not recommend the addition of a barrier. If not enough time is allowed for it to melt, a spermicide may not be in position to act effectively. When using spermicides, you should read the directions carefully and use the products exactly as directed! Remember, spermicidals alone are not 100% effective and are not recommended for those who must avoid pregnancy.

Combination birth control pills (those containing the female hormones estrogen and progesterone) prevent ovulation. Progesterone-only pills and Norplant (progestin containing capsules which are inserted under the skin of the upper arm) can also prevent ovu-

Some women with lupus should avoid certain contraceptive methods.

lation, but not consistently. They thicken the cervical mucus so it is difficult for the sperm to get through and they also change the lining of the uterus, making it an unwelcome place for both the sperm and egg. It was previously thought that birth control pills ought not to be prescribed for women with lupus since they might aggravate the disease. This concern is no longer generally accepted although such hormones, which may increase blood clotting, are still not advised for those women with anticardiolipin antibodies or the lupus anticoagulant. (See Chapter 2 for a discussion of these blood factors.)

IUDs, made of plastic, or plastic and copper, must be inserted into the uterus by a health care provider. They create local irritation which kills sperm and prevents the fertilized egg from implanting in the uterus. IUDs can increase the risk of infection and often cause increased bleeding during menstrual periods. Women with lupus who have decreased platelets, are on blood thinning medicine like coumadin, or have any other tendency towards increased bleeding are usually advised not to use IUDs.

Fertility awareness is based upon the woman knowing when she is fertile. The couple avoids intercourse on those days. Some types of fertility awareness methods include: the calendar rhythm method, the temperature method and the cervical mucus method. Using any of these methods requires very careful record keeping and strict self control to avoid intercourse at the fertile times. Anxiety, stress, or illness can delay ovulation and change the woman's usual cycle. If a patient wishes to use a cycle-based method of birth control, she should seek the advice of a physician who is very well versed in this type of birth control. These methods are often used because of a couples' religious beliefs. Catholic hospitals may be a source of literature, medical advice, counselling and support groups concerning how to use these methods properly.

The calendar based rhythm method requires keeping a calendar record of bleeding through eight menstrual cycles. The fertile period which occurs between menstrual periods is estimated by a formula which takes into account the average number of days of bleeding.

The temperature method requires that a woman take her resting temperature, known as basal body temperature (BBT), for 3-4 months in order to determine when she ovulates. The temperature must be taken every morning before getting out of bed and before performing any other activity. Tiny variations in temperature must be noted, e.g. noting one tenth of a degree may be crucial to the success of this method. A BBT thermometer (approximately $10) should be used. This only records readings from 96 degrees to a 100 degrees Fahrenheit. Usually just before ovulation a woman's temperature drops a few fractions of a degree. After ovulation, there is a rise from four tenths to eight tenths of a degree which continues until the next menstrual period.

The cervical mucus method is based on the fact that both the amount and consistency of the cervical mucus changes during the fertile period. The production of large amounts of thick mucus signals the onset of a fertile period. Checking the mucus requires that the woman inspect the mucus which is discharged out of the vagina each day and that she record changes in amount and consistency throughout a month or more until a pattern is established. This method is complicated by the fact that the vaginal discharge is changed by the presence of seminal fluid (the fluid released from the male during intercourse), by vaginal creams and jellies, by douches, and by vaginal infections. Despite these problems, cervical mucus inspection has some advantages over other fertility awareness methods especially for women with irregular menstrual cycles. Finally, there is a "morning after" pill that is a contraceptive. If the egg has been fertilized by a sperm, the pill prevents attachment of the fertilized egg to the uterus. If given less than 72 hours after a single episode of intercourse and continued for the next 5 days, this method is very effective.

Women's magazines and periodicals often tout the virtues of certain birth control methods. Friends always have opinions. Choosing the best method for you, however, should be based on medical guidance from a doctor who has knowledge of both family planning and lupus, on effectiveness, on cost, and on a full understanding and acceptance by both partners.

CHAPTER 18. PREGNANCY

Ronald Wapner, MD

Most patients with lupus can anticipate an uncomplicated and successful pregnancy. However, some lupus patients will experience difficulties. The like-

The risk of miscarriage is increased in lupus.

lihood of certain of these can be predicted prior to pregnancy while others cannot. In general, pregnancy will not alter the long-term outlook for the woman with lupus and the frequency of lupus flares should not increase following pregnancy. While it had previously been thought that there might be an increased risk of lupus worsening after the birth of the baby, this presently is not thought to be true.

Patients with lupus have an increased occurrence of miscarriage or pregnancy loss and the presence of certain antibodies may be predictive of which patients may be at risk. In particular, the presence of anticardiolipin antibodies (also sometimes referred to as antiphospholipid antibodies) or the lupus anticoagulant increase the risk of both early pregnancy loss (miscar-riage or spontaneous

A pregnancy complication called preeclampsia mimics a lupus flare.

abortion) and stillbirth (the birth of a dead fetus). In many cases, this problem can be treated with medication and the pregnancy can be completed successfully. All women with lupus should be tested before pregnancy for the presence of these antibodies and the lupus anticoagulant so any problems can be anticipated.

Certain maternal complications occur more frequently in women with lupus. Preeclampsia is a pregnancy condition that appears to occur more commonly in patients with lupus and includes an increase in maternal blood pressure, protein in the urine, and excessive retention of fluid (leg swelling, etc.). This appears to be most frequent in women whose kidneys are affected by lupus. Since the symptoms of preeclampsia are quite similar to those of a lupus flare, it is sometimes difficult to be certain which problem is occurring. This distinction is important since a lupus flare would be treated with steroids, while preeclampsia is managed with bed rest and is cured by delivery of the infant. In a small percentage of cases, preeclampsia becomes very severe in early pregnancy and premature delivery is necessary. However, the majority of patients developing this complication are able to carry the pregnancy long enough to allow fetal survival and excellent neonatal outcome. Most other complications of lupus such as arthritis, fatigue, skin rash, etc. do not present a problem during pregnancy. Patients with lupus involving either their lungs or their heart may have a special risk during pregnancy and should discuss this with their physician prior to conception.

A small group of infants born to mothers with lupus have the "neonatal lupus syndrome". This is usually a mild, short-lived condition though a few infants may require a pacemaker for an abnormal heartbeat (complete heart block) and some of these may not survive. (Neonatal lupus is discussed further in Chapter 15 on Childhood Disease.) Neonatal lupus is caused by certain of the mother's own abnormal antibodies (anti-Ro, also called anti-SSA; and anti-La also called anti-SSB) which cross the placenta to affect the fetus. For that reason, if a man with lupus fathers a child, his antibodies can not cause this kind of lupus in the infant.

Many medications required for the treatment of lupus have been utilized frequently during pregnancy and are generally felt to be safe. The use of steroids such as prednisone does not increase the risk of having a child with a birth defect but may present a slight increased risk of premature rupture of the membranes (the water bag breaking early). Low dose aspirin therapy has been shown to improve pregnancy outcome for patients at risk for miscarriage or fetal loss secondary to anticardiolipin antibodies. These low doses, usually only one baby aspirin per

Corticosteroids are generally safe for use during pregnancy.

day, will not cause fetal harm nor increase the risk of maternal complications. This dose of aspirin may also prevent occurrence of preeclampsia. Other nonsteroidal anti-inflammatory agents have also been utilized in pregnancy and like steroids have not been shown to increase the risk of birth defects. However, the use of these drugs later in pregnancy, usually after the completion of the seventh month, may affect the function of the fetal heart and blood vessels and, therefore, should not be used. Other medications such as Imuran and Plaquenil have been used successfully during pregnancy but the experience is more limited.

Labor and delivery are not usually altered for women with lupus although there is a slight increased risk of requiring a cesarean section. All forms of obstetric anesthesia can be utilized. The postpartum period and parenting should be uneventful. Women with lupus can breast-feed without any increased difficulties or risk to the infant. While some of the medications used to treat lupus may be present in the breast milk, this rarely causes a problem for the child since the level is low. The pediatrician should be aware of the use of these medications and can help decide whether breast-feeding is advisable.

Overall, most women with lupus can anticipate having children. However, it is strongly suggested that, prior to conceiving, they discuss their specific situations with an perinatologist (an obstetrician who specializes in high-risk pregnancy). It is usually preferable to plan a pregnancy while the lupus is in a quiescent state. While many patients can be cared for throughout pregnancy by their primary

Breast-feeding is safe for many women with lupus.

obstetrician along with their rheumatologist, some who have complications such as serious kidney disease or the presence of unusual antibodies may require the care of a perinatologist and delivery in a special center for high-risk cases.

CHAPTER 19. SOURCES OF SUPPORT

Carolyn H. McGrory, MS, RN

A chronic illness such as lupus affects not only people who have it, but also their families, their friends, their community and their work and schoolmates. At times this widening circle can include nearly anyone with whom they come in contact. The increasing involvement by others in their personal lives can sometimes be overwhelming. Looking at it from a positive point of view, it can also mean that there may be endless sources of support available. These may range from more traditional such as family, friends or churches, to increasingly popular "support groups".

> **People have a wonderful ability to help one another.**

What are support groups? Mutual support groups are available for nearly every problem imaginable. One city newspaper now has an entire half page devoted to support group

> **A shared problem is a less frightening problem.**

meeting times and places. The reason for this is clear: people – just ordinary people – have a wonderful ability to reach out to help one another and to draw strength from each other. Who better understands the problems you face with lupus and what is happening to your body than others who have had these or similar problems? When people have been through a series of lupus flares and remissions, they begin to recognize what helps and what doesn't. The support group provides a place to share this information and learn from one another. People who attend are often amazed at how creative they can be as they develop more and more insight into living with and coping with lupus.

What can you get from a support group? Perhaps the greatest benefit is total acceptance of yourself, just as you are. Sometimes people with lupus experience bizarre symptoms which come and go, seemingly with no reason. When they try to talk about these unusual complaints, they are often told that the problems are all "in their heads". As a result, they begin to lose self-confidence and start to question whether or not they have imagined the problems. When a support group member gathers up his or her courage to mention such things (occasional episodes of short-term memory loss, for example), imagine how relieved he or she feels to look up and see fourteen other nodding heads. A problem that has been experienced and acknowledged by others somehow becomes less frightening. Other common problems, such as coping with overwhelming fatigue or living with the terrible uncertainty of never knowing how you will feel tomorrow, can be shared safely in a support group.

Some people are skeptical about attending a group session. They say that they don't want to sit around and hear a lot of "sick people" complain. The truth is, there may be a lot of sick people in attendance but they are not just sitting around complaining. There is joy, acceptance, trust and help in this group where people have the courage to be honest and truly care about one another. A facilitator of a lupus support group once remarked that her more than ten-year contact with that group was one of the most enriching of her life. Those sentiments are probably typical of the positive influence many support groups have.

Now how about your family and friends – what can they gain from being a part of a support group? It's a funny thing about families and friends. Sometimes they are so close to you that, as the saying goes, they "cannot see the forest for the trees". They lose their ability to be objective. They love you and they hate that you are sick. Sometimes their anger at the disease may seem to be directed at you personally. They, like you, may feel helpless and hopeless, even though they don't actually experience exactly what you are going through. When they hear concerns and symptoms similar to yours from a normal-appearing stranger, it can help them to begin to understand and communicate with you in a new and more appropriate way.

What if there is no support group nearby? Our suggestion is to start one. A mutual support group, by definition, is one which evolves from, and revolves around, those who share a com-

If no support group exists, start one.

mon concern. Find each other – from the doctor's office or the local lupus foundation or by means of an advertisement placed in the newspaper. Plan a time and a date, and then meet. The group can be as organized as you wish – either formally, with elected officers and a specific topic for discussion, or casually, sharing a cup of tea and discussing whatever comes up. A group can be very successful, but there are also potential pitfalls. People with lupus know that there is always the possibility of being too sick or too fatigued or just not feeling able when the time comes to attend the meeting. It may sometimes be difficult, therefore, for a person with lupus either to lead or to participate in a support group on a regular basis. Stay flexible and don't be discouraged if attendance in the group varies from time to time. If you cannot do it alone, another option is to enlist a health professional (such as a physical therapist, nurse, social worker, occupational therapist, or psychologist) to help with the group and act as facilitator. An added benefit of this approach is that many health professionals are associated with institutions which have meeting rooms and publicity departments that can be used by the group. Since lupus is such a varied and sometimes confusing disease, it may also be important to have a health professional there as a resource to provide up-to-date and accurate information. You can find an appropriate person through your doctor's office, the local hospital or other health care facility. Whichever way you choose to start your group, it takes time to get a support group going, so don't give up.

What is the bottom line about support? Not everyone has a family or appropriate friends or a handy support group. You may have to look in the mirror and decide that the bottom line is YOU. You may find that you want to deny the very existence of your lupus. Eventually, however, you must face the reality of living and coping with it. Occasionally, you must give yourself permission to be afraid, to be sad, and to be angry. If you are becoming depressed, seek psychological help early. When flares come, you will have to reassess yourself and temporarily accommodate to your changed condition. When they

What can be positive about having lupus?

pass, go back to living your life to the fullest that your personal experience with lupus will allow. Gather all the help you can from doctors, nurses, social workers and therapists. Remember that you have the right to total information about the disease, about your condition and about possible treatments. Seek guidance and information from your local lupus foundation chapter. Live as healthy a life style as possible. Learn about proper nutrition, the best way to exercise when you have a chronic illness, and methods to help you conserve energy on those days when fatigue may be overwhelming. Ask questions, take notes and make your own decisions.

Try to focus on the positives in life from among the negatives of having a chronic illness like lupus. A few years ago one of our colleagues conducted a study of 125 people with lupus. She asked them if there was anything positive about having the disease. To her surprise nearly everyone said "yes". Lupus had given them the chance to value those things in life which they had formerly taken for granted. These included really enjoying each healthy day, improving their relationship with God, and finding great pleasure in simple things such as watching the sunset. Chronic illness may take its toll physically and emotionally, but it also enables you to recognize just what an exceptional person you are – a person who can develop and work toward new goals and expectations, those that not only accommodate to living with lupus but also enhance life itself.

Chapter 20.   The Doctor-Patient Relationship

Mary E. Moore, PhD, MD

(In an attempt to make this chapter more readable, we will arbitrarily refer to the patient as "she" and the doctor as "he". We hope the reader [she or he] will forgive us this generalization.)

The doctor-patient relationship is one of the most important factors determining successful treatment of a chronic disease. Patients with lupus often face special problems which can greatly influence this relationship. Lupus patients may require years of continual care and, since lupus in-

The last decade has brought great changes to medical care delivery.

volves many body systems, they may require the services of several doctors at the same time. Lupus is not well understood by many members of the medical profession, and since there is a lot about lupus that remains unknown even to experts, patients may encounter varying degrees of ignorance about their disease. Finally, since lupus has psychological as well as physical effects, lupus patients often experience difficulties with interpersonal interactions. These may carry over into the doctor-patient relationship.

The traditional doctor-patient relationship has changed in the United States over the last decade.

The previous model of interaction between patient and physician was based on the fact that the patient was free to choose a physician who, in turn, could expect to be reimbursed for the specific service rendered. This model holds now for a shrinking proportion of the population and several quite different models are becoming increasingly widespread. Currently, the government is addressing the question of how to assure that its citizens get good quality, affordable medical care. Many people have expressed the fear that a new government-sponsored plan will change the doctor-patient relationship. It is important to recognize, however, that even if the government fails to make any changes, the high cost of modern medical care is such that employers and insurance companies have already modified, and will continue to modify, the way in which that care is delivered. As a result, many aspects of the doctor-patient relationship have already been affected.

The most radical changes in the doctor-patient relationship have occurred in the setting of health maintenance organizations (HMOs) in which, at present, almost 70 million Americans are enrolled. In a typical HMO, a primary care doctor (usually a general or a family practitioner, a general internist, or – sometimes in the case of a woman patient – a gynecologist) acts as a "gatekeeper". He makes a contract with a medical insurance company to care for a number of patients for a certain period of time for a fixed fee. When a

A typical HMO pays a doctor a fixed fee to care for a patient.

patient who is a member of an HMO visits the primary care doctor, she pays nothing or only a token fee. If the patient needs more specialized care, the referral for that care has to be approved by the primary care doctor and the specialist's fee is paid by the insurance company from a special fund. If at the end of a certain time period, there is money remaining in that fund, it is awarded to the primary care physician. Thus the primary care physician makes more money when the patient is healthier and does not require the care of specialists. Such a system works very well for healthy people, especially those with children who can thus afford preventive care for their families. It works less well for people with a complicated chronic illness such as lupus.

Other systems of healthcare delivery combine aspects of the traditional system and elements of an HMO system with innovations of their own. Some HMOs hire physicians and pay them a salary. Some physicians and hospitals band together to provide inexpensive care in a Preferred Provider Organization (PPO). The PPO then contracts with an employer who requires that their employees receive all of their medical care from that PPO. All insurers limit, much more closely than in the past, expensive forms of treatment. As a result, some decisions regarding patient care which were once made by the doctor and the patient are now, for all practical purposes, being made by insurers.

Insurers make some decisions formerly made by doctors and patients.

With all of these changes, it is incumbent upon the patient to assume much more responsibility for her own care than was necessary in years past. This task is made easier if one understands some basic elements of the doctor-patient relationship.

Doctors And Patients Approach Illness Differently

The doctor's primary goal is to arrive at the correct diagnosis and to arrange for appropriate treatment. A secondary goal is to end the patient's fear and suffering, if possible. Patients hope, above all, to have their fear and suffering alleviated. They also hope that any treatment will be as painless and as harmless as possible.

In the case of lupus, the problem of diagnosis may be a major one. Most physicians do not see many cases of lupus and may have difficulty recognizing it. In early cases, even experienced rheumatologists (doctors who specialize in the rheumatic diseases) at times do not agree on the diagnosis. Physicians are reluctant to label anyone as having a serious disease until they are certain of the diagnosis. They may order a number of tests before committing themselves to a diagnosis and thus inadvertently add to the patient's feelings of uncertainty. While the doctor attempts to verify the diagnosis, patients, unaware of the doctor's goal, may feel that not enough attention is being given to their specific complaints and fears.

Problems can also arise between the doctor and the patient with lupus over the issue of treatment. The physician may feel that because the patient's lupus has caused potentially life-threatening complications, it is necessary to prescribe steroids or immunosuppressive drugs such as those used in the chemotherapy of cancer. Such treatments have undesirable and dangerous side effects which must be explained to patients but which may frighten them and cause them to refuse treatment. The resulting discussion may frustrate the doctor and cause the patient to question whether the doctor has her best interests at heart.

Some Things The Patient Should Expect From The Doctor:

- That the doctor is well-trained and competent to practice medicine.
- That the doctor is a responsible person who will live up to his obligations, and always try his best.
- That the doctor will seek help from others if he reaches the limits of his knowledge or ability and will communicate willingly and fully with any consultant if requested to do so by the patient.
- That the doctor is of good moral character, and will never take advantage of the physical intimacy which the patient must permit.
- That the doctor will hold in confidence any personal information disclosed and will not release information to anyone concerning the patient without the patient's permission.
- That the doctor will treat the patient with respect and courtesy and will display concern about the suffering and fears of the patient.

- That the doctor will make a continuing effort to explain to the patient the nature of the illness and its treatment.
- That the doctor will arrange for suitable coverage when he is not available.

Since lupus is a relatively unusual disorder and may be very difficult to manage, patients with lupus must be certain that their doctor is qualified by training and experience to treat their disease. An internist, one who has completed residency training in internal medicine, is often the type of physician called upon to provide primary care for lupus. Board certification in Internal Medicine (the physician will probably display the certificate in his office) is one indication of good training. In addition, it is quite appropriate for patients to ask the doctor how much experience he has had with lupus.

The patient with lupus should expect that the doctor will freely entertain requests for second opinions. These opinions may be needed when the diagnosis is in question or when a change of treatment is contemplated. A rheumatologist is usually the most knowledgeable specialist to consult concerning diagnosis or general treatment of lupus (and, under some types of insurance may provide primary care for lupus patients). Dermatologists are frequently consulted concerning the diagnosis of lupus in patients whose illness is associated with skin changes.

Patients should also expect that their physicians will seek help from other specialists when complications develop. Examples of complications of lupus which often require the help of specialists are kidney failure, which may need the help of a nephrologist; seizures and strokes, which may call for the help of a neurologist; and inflammation of the lining or muscle of the heart, for which the advice of a cardiologist may be required.

The issue of obtaining second opinions or consultations with specialists may become a special issue for lupus patients enrolled in HMOs. It may become necessary for patients to insist on such referrals and to take special precautions when they are granted. Recent blood test results, x-rays, and biopsy slides are best hand-carried by the patient to assure they are available at the time the consultant is seen. It is also best to have a note from the referring doctor stating exactly what is being requested. Finally the HMO patient must have, at the time of the visit, a referral form signed by the referring physician stating the number of visits the referral permits and whether or not the consulting physician is authorized only to evaluate the patient or may perform any appropriate procedure (such as a biopsy or injection of a joint). If the doctor evaluates or treats the HMO patient without such a form, the HMO will not reimburse him for such services and may strike him from the list of potential consultants.

Some Things The Patient Should <u>Not</u> Expect From The Doctor:
- That the doctor can find a solution for every physical problem.
- That the doctor will treat the patient with the af-

fection of a close friend or family member.
- That the doctor is the patient's employee and will provide service on demand.
- That the doctor can always personally be available to the patient.
- That the doctor has unlimited time to spend with the patient.
- That medicine is an exact science and that every doctor will come to the same conclusions and recommendations when looking at the same set of medical problems.
- That the doctor can always make the layman understand very complex medical problems.

Patients with lupus must realize that they have a chronic disease for which there is no cure. Because the disease is life-long and because it can be very complex, the lupus patient who finds a good doctor will do well to stay with that doctor. Whenever patients switch doctors or change hospitals, vital information about their case may be distorted or lost. Information about the way the disease has affected the patient in the past is very important. Sometimes the key to understanding what is going on in lupus at any one time is to understand the pattern of previous flares of the disease.

Many lupus patients, like those with other chronic diseases, grow dependent on their physicians and look up to them as they would to parents or loving friends. Doctors, however, are not comfortable treating their own children or their good friends. Doctors must keep some distance between themselves and their patients so that their emotional response does not get in the way of their medical judgment. That's why doctors must set limits on the demands patients may make of them. Except for emergencies, doctors usually consult with patients only during office hours. They provide substitute physicians to cover their practice when they will not be available. Some of the most highly qualified doctors are affiliated with large teaching hospitals and often have young doctors in training (residents or fellows) helping them take care of patients.

A major source of confusion between a doctor and a patient with a complex condition such as lupus often centers around the doctor's attempts to explain the illness in everyday language. At times this may not be possible and the patient must be willing to trust the doctor's judgment even without fully understanding the reasoning behind it. Since information about lupus and even the words used to describe this information are constantly changing, no two doctors are likely to understand or explain lupus in exactly the same way. In addition, when physicians translate their understanding from medical to everyday vocabulary, they may do so in different ways. The patient with lupus commonly hears different explanations of a problem from different doctors. For example, one doctor may explain that lupus is the result of the body's defenses attacking itself, that lupus is an autoimmune disease. Another may describe lupus as an inflammation of blood vessels known as vasculitis. Still a third may say that lupus is a connective tissue disease somewhat similar to rheumatoid arthritis. All are correct.

Some Things The Doctor Should Expect From The Patient:

- That within the limits of the patient's ability, she will be responsible for knowing her past medical history and treatment.
- That the patient will not hide facts about her illness.
- That the patient will try to follow the doctor's suggestions for treatment, or will inform the doctor when this has not been done.
- That the patient will keep her appointments, or will cancel as soon as possible those which cannot be kept.
- That the patient will treat the doctor courteously and politely.
- That the patient will take responsibility to ask questions about those parts of her illness and its treatment that she does not understand well.
- That the patient will not ask the doctor to act illegally or unethically.
- That the patient or a third party such as an insurance carrier will pay the doctor for his services.

Patients with lupus can be most helpful by keeping records of major medical events with notes about what medications have been taken, what doses were used, when they were begun, and how long they were taken. Such records are especially important when the patient takes steroids. The patient's pattern of using these drugs can provide valuable clues about the disease activity. Patients who have been on steroids for a long time sometimes increase the dose on their own when they feel ill or may forget to take medication when they feel well. If this happens, the doctor must be told so he can prescribe future medication correctly.

Physicians cannot be expected to make false statements to benefit the patient on prescriptions, insurance or disability forms no matter how trivial these may seem. Not only does such behavior compromise the physician's ethical standards, it can potentially lead to loss of his medical license.

HMO patients or those with similar medical plans which limit the doctor's reimbursement cannot expect to receive treatment which is not covered or authorized. New questions about illness which arise between visits should ordinarily be addressed to the primary physician who is being reimbursed to provide continuing care for the patient.

Some Things The Doctor Should Not Expect From The Patient:

- That the patient will be grateful to the doctor for her care.
- That the patient will never question the doctor's opinion.
- That the patient will unquestioningly follow the doctor's medical orders.
- That the patient will always be able to keep anger, depression or fear concerning her illness under control and will never displace it onto the doctor.
- That the patient will share the same moral customs and values as the doctor.
- That the patient has any obligation to continue under the doctor's care.

Physicians who treat patients with lupus must be very careful not to interpret patients' emotional response to their illness as a reflection of their feelings about their physician. Lupus patients are sometimes angry or depressed. The doctor must learn not to feel threatened by such emotions but must try to determine their cause. They may result from, or may be made worse by, effects of medication such as steroids or they may be the result of activity of the lupus itself.

The physician must also be on guard not to allow generational and cultural gaps to widen the distance between doctor and patient. For example, studies done in a variety of medical settings show that male physicians sometimes discount the complaints of female patients to a greater extent than they would do those of male patients.

In Conclusion

Many patients are disappointed because they expect their doctor to be a combination of parent, friend, and miracle worker and they blame him for things which are beyond his control. Others are unhappy because they fail to understand the extent to which they must assume responsibility for their own medical care. Many doctors are unhappy because they expect patients to follow orders without question, to be undemanding, and never to succumb to fear or anger. Some are frustrated because they feel their authority is being diminished by changes in the system of medical care delivery. Hopefully, if the parties involved in the doctor-patient relationship could look at this interaction more objectively and each could consider the viewpoint of the other, it would be to the mutual advantage of both.

Chapter 21. Answers To Commonly Asked Questions

Sheldon Solomon, MD

Q: **Is lupus a fatal disease?**

A: No. The life expectancy of people with SLE has improved steadily. This is partly due to earlier diagnosis and, partly, to improvement in treatment. In a study done in 1989 almost 9 out of 10 people with SLE were still alive 10 years after their diagnosis. If such a study were done today, this number would probably be even higher.

Q: **Is lupus catching?**

A: Lupus is not infectious. You cannot "catch" it from any kind of close contact. When a family member of a lupus patient gets lupus, we believe that is because he or she has some inherited tendency in common and may have met up with the same, or some other, "trigger" of the disease. A "trigger" is something in the environment that can set off the disease in people who, because of their inheritance, are prone to get it.

Q: **I have discoid lupus. What are the chances of my developing systemic lupus erythematosus?**

A: Discoid lupus involves having a certain kind of chronic rash most often on the face, scalp, ears or neck – the vast majority of people who have this form of lupus have only skin involvement. Only about one in ten people with discoid lupus will go on to develop systemic lupus erythematosus. Those who have discoid lupus with a rash which is widespread, involving areas of the body below the neck and the arms and legs, have a greater chance of developing systemic lupus erythematosus than those whose discoid rash is confined to the face and head.

Q: **I have lupus. What chance is there that my children will get it?**

A: There does seem to be a genetic basis to lupus – for example, if one identical twin has it, there is a slightly better than a 50-50 chance of the other twin developing it. However, the chance of a child of a mother with lupus coming down with the disease is very slim – only about 2 or 3 chances in 100.

Q: **Should lupus patients receive flu shots?**

A: Patients with lupus have a greater susceptibility to infections in general compared to healthy people. This is particularly so in those lupus patients on corticosteroids or immunosuppressive drugs. For this reason it is generally recommended that lupus patients have a flu shot annually, although the final decision would rest with the patient and his or her own physician. Lupus patients also have an increased risk of pneumococcal pneumonia and they should probably receive the vaccination (Pneumovax) against this also. This is given only once every 6 years.

Q: **Why is it so difficult to make a diagnosis of lupus?**

A: There is no one simple test that will make a diagnosis of SLE. The diagnosis is made when a combination of problems (arthritis, rash, fever, kidney problems, pleurisy, etc.) occur along with abnormal blood test results such as a positive antinuclear antibody, an ANA. Often, in early SLE, only a few problems such as fever, fatigue or achiness are present. These might suggest a host of other diseases and so a definite diagnosis cannot be made at that time. Watching and waiting to see what will develop, at the same time trying to relieve the patient's symptoms, is the only thing that can be done

Q: **My doctor says my lupus is in remission. Does that mean that I don't have the disease any more?**

A: Patients with lupus have their "ups" and "downs." At times the disease may flare and be very active; at other times it may appear to be gone or in remission. However the genetic predisposition that led to the disease developing in the first place is still present. The disease is never really ever gone permanently. In lupus brought on by certain drugs, however, removing the offending drug (Pronestyl, Apresoline, etc.) can end the disease.

Q: **How can I tell if my lupus is sun sensitive and what do I do if it is?**

A: The most common manifestation of sun sensitivity is the sudden development of a rash, usually involving the cheeks and nose (the butterfly pattern) shortly after sitting in the sun or attending a tanning parlor. Occasionally other symptoms such as fever, joint pains or fatigue may occur after such exposure. If you are a newly diagnosed patient with lupus and are not sure whether you are sun sensitive it is probably wise to be extremely careful in the sun. You should use a good sunscreen (sun protection factor of at least 15). It must be placed on all sun exposed areas of the skin one half hour before going into the sun. It should be reapplied if you get wet or perspire heavily. It is best to avoid sun exposure between 10:00 A.M. and 4:00 P.M. Protective clothing with long sleeves and wide brimmed hats should be worn.

Q: **I am a woman with lupus who has taken steroids for eleven years and am concerned about osteoporosis. What are the pros and cons of estrogen replacement?**

A: Steroids, (prednisone, Medrol, etc.) injure bone by removing calcium and by preventing calcium taken by mouth from being absorbed. For this reason, high dosages of calcium along with an adequate amount of vitamin D, which is necessary for calcium absorption, should be taken to prevent osteoporosis. You should also realize that smoking cigarettes, drinking alcohol to excess, and living a very sedentary life-style can increase osteoporosis and you should try to correct these problems. Estrogen is very helpful in preventing calcium loss from bones and also protects against some types of heart disease. High levels of a hormone related to estrogen are seen in lupus patients and women, who have more estrogen than men, get lupus more often than men. Nevertheless, it is not thought that taking estrogen replacement has any adverse effect on lupus. But estrogen is not recommended for women with a history of breast cancer or those who have close blood relatives with it and estrogen increases the risk of cancer of the uterus. So, the question of whether you should use estrogen replacement must be given some thought and decided in consultation with your doctor.

Q: **I take Plaquenil. Is my eyesight in danger?**

A: Plaquenil in doses used today to treat lupus carries a very low risk of damaging eyesight. Check-ups every 6 months with an ophthalmologist can uncover early changes. If such changes are seen, stopping the drug can minimize this very rare chance of losing eyesight.

Q: **Can I do anything to lessen the side effects of prednisone? The weight gain, the facial puffiness, the muscle cramps, and the thinning of bone?**

A: In lupus patients taking prednisone, certain dietary

modifications are in order. First a low calorie diet is mandatory. Prednisone increases appetite so that this may be difficult. You should drink plenty of water and eat lots of vegetables such as tomatoes, carrots, celery, etc. These are low calorie and filling. You should adhere to a low-salt diet, avoiding the salt shaker and salty foods such as pretzels and potato chips. Foods high in calcium and low in fat such as skim milk and low-fat yogurt are recommended to strengthen bone without increasing cholesterol. Foods high in potassium such as citrus fruits and bananas will help lessen the muscle cramps.

Q: **What drugs are used to treat the kidney involvement in lupus?**

A: Prednisone is commonly used. The dose and the length of treatment depend on the severity of the kidney disease. Other drugs that are used with prednisone, or in place of it, are the immunosuppressive drugs Imuran and Cytoxan.

Q: **What does having a positive ANA mean?**

A: Often not very much. It may be positive in patients treated with certain drugs including some heart, blood pressure and seizure medication. The ANA may be weakly positive in ten to twenty percent of completely normal people. The test may be positive in patients with many other connective tissue diseases such as rheumatoid arthritis. It may be positive in a host of other diseases such as hepatitis, Lyme disease, certain heart infections (endocarditis), and thyroid disease. After the ANA is determined to be positive, the titer of ANA is determined. A titer is a measure of the relative amount of something which is present. In the case of ANA, a titer is a way of saying that the ANA is weakly or strongly positive. To figure the titer of an ANA, the patient's serum, that part of the blood which contains the ANA, is diluted with more and more of a neutral fluid to see if the positive ANA still shows up. If the ANA still shows up as positive after the serum is diluted with the same volume of the neutral fluid, the titer of ANA is said to be 1:2. If the positive ANA persists when the serum is diluted with twice as much neutral fluid, the titer is said to be 1:3. A titer of ANA equal to or greater than 1:80 is the number considered meaningful by most rheumatologists. To be useful, a positive ANA test result must be consistent with the information the physician obtains during his examination of the patient. ANA tests are often of most value when results are negative, since a negative test almost always means the patient does not have lupus.

Q: **What is a sedimentation rate and what does it mean if it is elevated?**

A: The sedimentation rate, sometimes called the erythrocyte sedimentation rate or the ESR, is a simple inexpensive test that involves measuring how fast the patient's red blood cells settle to the bottom of a special glass tube. The test results are given in terms of millimeters per hour. The higher the number, the faster the cells have settled. The numbers for males are normally lower than those for females. The ESR is a crude measure of the amount of inflammatory protein in the blood. It is not specific for lupus and sometimes corresponds poorly with disease activity in lupus.

Q: **My family doesn't understand how tired and weak my lupus makes me feel. What can I do to make them understand?**

A: You and your family would benefit greatly by joining a lupus support group. There your family can see that other lupus patients have the same complaints you do. They can also see that they are not alone in having difficultly coping with a family member when he or she is sick. You can inquire about a support group near you by calling your local Lupus Foundation, the Arthritis Foundation or the national Lupus Foundation of America at 1-800-558-0121.

Q: **What are anticardiolipin antibodies and what does it mean if you have them?**

A: These are a group of antibodies that are sometimes found in lupus patients as well as in others who do not have lupus. These antibodies are associated with blood clots in arteries and veins and with miscarriages. If you have the antibody present and have had no trouble as a result, then your doctor might recommend you take one baby aspirin a day to prevent problems. If you have the antibody and have had a stroke, or a miscarriage, or a blood clot in your leg, you will probably require life-long thinning of the blood with a drug called coumadin.

Q: **What are the side effects of Cytoxan?**

A: Cytoxan is one of the immunosuppressant drugs used in lupus to overcome serious disease. It is also widely used in the treatment of cancer. It has many potential side effects and careful monitoring by a physician well versed in using the drug is recommended. Nausea and vomiting is occasionally seen when it is given by mouth and used to be encountered quite often when it was given by vein. Now, however, a drug called Zofran given along with intravenous Cytoxan dramatically reduces vomiting. Loss of scalp hair sometimes occurs with Cytoxan. The hair usually grows back when treatment is stopped. Blood counts must be checked while taking Cytoxan because in some doses it can affect the bone marrow and prevent formation of white or red cells and platelets leading to susceptibility to infections, anemia, and bleeding problems. Cytoxan may cause a failure to menstruate and poor sperm formation. It should never be taken if pregnancy is feasible because of the possibility of birth defects. Cytoxan also irritates the bladder and bleeding into the urine can result. Scar tissue can build up in the bladder and may lead to bladder cancer. There is also a small but definite increase of other types of cancer in patients taking long-term Cytoxan.

Q: **Should I stop taking prednisone and Plaquenil if I become pregnant?**

A: First of all, never stop prednisone abruptly without first talking to your physician. This can cause a flare of your disease or may even cause shock. Prednisone may be continued during pregnancy if required to control lupus since it has not been associated with abnormalities in the developing fetus. It is also probably safe to continue Plaquenil during pregnancy. Because of the potential of birth defects, other drugs such as methotrexate, Imuran, and Cytoxan are not advisable, if they are not essential, if there is any chance that you might become pregnant.

Q: **I have dizzy spells and memory loss. Could this be lupus affecting the brain?**

A: Lupus can affect the entire nervous system, including the brain, spinal cord, and the nerves to all parts of the body. Memory loss and dizzy spells could be due to lupus. However, not everything that bothers you is lupus. Memory loss and dizzy spells are very non-specific and could be entirely unrelated to lupus. Both could arise from the stress you experience living with this chronic disease. Many medications could contribute to the memory loss, such as tranquilizers, blood pressure medicines and sleeping pills. It would be wise to discuss these symptoms with your physician.

Q: **I never seem to get my questions answered when I see my doctor and I'm not sure who is**

at fault. What do you think?

A: It would be a good idea for you to make a list of questions before seeing your doctor. After you have answered the doctor's questions about how you are feeling and after doctor's examination, inquire if there is time for you to ask the questions on your list. Because the doctor has other patients scheduled, you may need to set up a special appointment just directed to answering your questions.

Q: **My cousin has Lyme disease but for about six months was told it was lupus. Why is this?**

A: Both of these diseases share many things in common including arthritis, fatigue, rash, nerve irritation. It often is difficult to decide which is which. Even the laboratory tests for one or the other may be misleading. For example, patients with lupus may have a "positive" test for Lyme; the opposite being true also – patients with Lyme also may have a "positive" ANA. People like your cousin would do best to consult a rheumatologist, a doctor who specializes in both diseases and understands the difficulties of interpreting test results.

Q: **I have been sick with lupus for over ten years. At present I have four different doctors taking care of me. Couldn't I just go to one doctor?**

A: It is very difficult for any one physician to care for such a complex disease as lupus. Your general internist, your primary care physician or your rheumatologist may centralize your care but may need help, for example, from the ophthalmologist who checks for eye toxicity from drugs like prednisone and Plaquenil, the nephrologist who does a kidney biopsy and supervises dialysis, the orthopedic surgeon who performs surgery on damaged joints, etc.

Q: **A friend of mine who has lupus told me she feels great since she began to take vitamins and other preparations from the health food store. What do you think?**

A: Vitamins and minerals are occasionally needed in the sick patient with lupus who is not eating a balanced diet. In general, however, vitamins and minerals belong to a long list of products that we call unproven remedies. There are no scientific data showing they work to cure lupus and neither is there any showing that they are harmful. A problem with unproven remedies is that their manufacture is often not well controlled. A recent example of problems in manufacture was provided by the discovery of cases of muscle damage brought on by contaminated tryptophan, a substance sold in health food stores to promote sleep. Certainly before trying unproven remedies, you should discuss them with your physician.

Q: **What is fibromyalgia? I've heard that it might be difficult to tell the difference between it and lupus?**

A: Fibromyalgia is a condition that causes widespread stiffness and pain centered around the neck and upper arms, and the back and upper legs. It results in a number of specific tender points, the presence of which help the doctor to diagnosis the condition. No laboratory tests are positive in fibromyalgia and experts disagree concerning whether we should think of it as a real disease. People who have lupus sometimes get symptoms of fibromyalgia. They may be said to have secondary fibromyalgia. People with fibromyalgia sometimes worry that they might have lupus. Lupus is always diagnosed as discussed in Chapters 1 and 3, however, and there should never be great difficulty in deciding whether someone has lupus or simple fibromyalgia.

INDEX

A

abdominal pain 6, 23, 46
acetaminophen 127
acne 137
active assisted range of motion 144
activities of daily living 148
Advil 24, 48, 134. *See also* ibuprofen
age 83
AIDS 157
AJAO (American Juvenile Arthritis
  Organization) 137
alcohol 114, 116, 191
alendronate 115
Aleve 24, 48. *See also* ibuprofen
alfalfa seeds 44
alopecia 5. *See also* hair
American College of Rheumatology
  (ACR) 3, 132
American Heart Association 122
ANA. *See* antinuclear antibody (ANA)
Anaprox 24
anemia 4, 7, 35, 53, 55, 103, 195
anemia of chronic disease 104
anemia of kidney disease 105
anti-ds (double-stranded) DNA
  antibodies 30
anti-Jo-1 antibodies 33
anti-La antibodies 165
anti-oxidant vitamins 96
anti-PM 1 antibodies 33
anti-RNP (ribonucleoprotein)
  antibodies 31
anti-Ro (or SS-A) antibodies 31, 139,
  165
anti-Sm (Smith) antibodies 31
antibodies 108
anticardiolipin antibodies 32, 73, 160,
  163, 194
anticentromere antibodies 33
anticonvulsant medication 73
antihistone antibodies 31
antimalarial drugs 48, 61, 100, 135
antineuronal antibodies 73
antinuclear antibody (ANA) 8, 27, 38
antiphospholipid antibodies 163
antiphospholipid syndrome 21, 32, 75,
  109, 128, 149

antiribosomal P protein antibodies 73
antiscleroderma 70 (anti-Scl-70)
  antibodies 32
anxiety 74, 85, 89
Apresoline 189
Aralen 48
arthritis 4, 5, 8, 154
Arthritis Foundation 137, 156, 194
artificial saliva 127
Ascriptin 24. *See also* aspirin
aspirin 21, 46, 48, 127, 134, 165
Atabrine 48
atherosclerosis 52
attention 82
autoantibodies 30
autoimmune hemolytic anemia 106
avascular necrosis 5, 52, 111, 115, 117
azathioprine (Imuran) 53, 61, 135

B

B lymphocytes 108
bad breath 125
band test 62
barrier contraceptives 158
basal body temperature (BBT) 161
beta carotene 97
biologicals 55
birth control pills 160
birth defect 165
bite-guard 127
bleeding 109
blood 103–109
blood clots 21
blood pressure 65, 75, 76, 87
bone 111–119
bone marrow 7, 53, 65, 104, 105, 108,
  195
boys 131
brain 72, 79, 86, 99, 141
brain dysfunction 82
breast-feed 166
butterfly rash 4, 61

C

calcitonin 114
calcium 45, 114, 190, 192

J

Jaccoud's arthropathy 14
joint replacement 149
joints 13, 141
judgement 82
juvenile rheumatoid arthritis 132

K

K-Y jelly 154
ketoprofen 48
kidney 6, 9, 34, 45, 46, 55, 65–70, 105,
    135, 192
kidney biopsy 67, 133
kidney disorders 50
kidney transplant 68
knee 147

L

laboratory tests 27–35
language skills 82
lens 94, 95
Leukeran 53
leukocytes 35
libido 155
Librium 89
life expectancy 187
lips 124
livedo reticularis 5, 21
liver 132
"Living and Loving with Arthritis" 155
low density lipoprotein (LDL) 19
lungs 22
lupus anticoagulant 32, 75, 160
Lupus Foundation of America 194
Lyme disease 132, 192, 197
lymph nodes 25
lymphocytes 1, 7, 108

M

magnetic resonance imaging (MRI) 34
malaise 43
malar 61
management 43
Masters and Johnson 159
Medi-Alert bracelet 51
medical profession 173
medications 45. *See also* individual
    drugs

Medrol 50, 135, 155, 190
memory 82, 87, 196
meningitis 76
menstrual cycle 137
menstruation 132
mental illness 74
methotrexate 14, 53, 157
methyldopa 10
methylprednisolone 50
miscarriages 32, 138, 195
misoprostol 25, 157
mixed connective tissue disease 8
molecular biology 39
mononeuritis 76
mood 88, 133
morning after pill 158, 162
motor performance 82
Motrin 24, 48, 134
MRI (magnetic resonance imaging) 77,
    118, 133
muscles 13, 15
myocarditis 17
myositis 76

N

Naprosyn 24, 134
naproxen 24, 48, 134
neonatal lupus 139, 164
nephritis 132
nephrologist 179, 198
nephrotic syndrome 66
nerve conduction study 77
nervous system 71
neuro-ophthalmologist 99
neurologist 71, 133, 179
neuropsychologist 81
nonsteroidal anti-inflammatory drugs
    (NSAIDS) 24, 46, 76, 105, 122,
    134
Norplant implants 158, 159
numerical abilities 82
Nuprin 24, 48
nurse 136, 170
nutrition 44

O

obstetrician 156, 166
occupational therapist 142, 170
Office of Vocational Rehabilitation
    (OVR) 136

ophthalmologist 101
optic nerve 94
oral contraceptives 138
oral ulcers 5, 153
organic brain syndrome 73
orthopedic surgeon 148, 198
Orudis KT 48
osteoarthritis 117
osteoporosis 52, 111, 112, 114, 147, 190
osteotomy 118
ovulation 161

P

pacemaker 139, 165
paralysis 75, 141
passive range of motion 144
patients 173
pediatrician 166
penis 62
perception 82
Percocet 113
pericarditis 6, 16, 22, 24, 46, 132
periodontal disease 122, 124
periodontitis 123
peripheral nerves 72, 74
peritoneal dialysis 69
peritonitis 6, 23
personality 74, 79, 82
pheresis 54
photosensitivity 59
physiatrist 142
physical therapist 142, 170
physician 43
plaque 125
Plaquenil 48, 76, 100, 135, 166, 191,
    196
plasmapheresis 54
platelets 4, 7, 21, 32, 35, 47, 53, 103,
    108, 160, 195
pleuritis 4, 6, 9, 22, 24, 46
pneumococcal pneumonia 188
pneumonitis 22
Pneumovax 26, 189
polarizing lenses 96
polymyositis 33
potassium 192
PPO 175
prednisolone 50. *See also* corticoster-
    oids
prednisone 111, 135, 155, 190, 191,
    196. *See also* corticosteroids

preeclampsia 164
Preferred Provider Organization (PPO)
    175
pregnancy 9, 21, 32, 132, 138, 156,
    163–167, 195
procainamide 10
progesterone 138, 159
Pronestyl 189
prophylactic antibiotics 122, 126
psychiatrist 133
psychologist 142, 143, 170
psychosis 88, 91
puberty 131, 137
pulmonary hypertension 23
pulse 51
pulse therapy 68

Q

quinacrine 48
quinidine 10

R

rash 132
Raynaud's phenomenon 19
reasoning 82
recreational therapist 142
red blood cells 103
referral form 179
rehabilitation 141–151
remission 189
residents 181
retina 49, 94, 98
rheumatic fever 132
rheumatoid arthritis 8, 14, 31, 192
rheumatoid factor 8, 33
rheumatologist 156, 176, 178, 198
Rheumatrex 53
rosacea 61

S

sadness 89
salt 45
school 135
scleroderma 8, 20, 31, 33
seborrheic dermatitis 61
sedentary life-style 191
sedimentation rate 193
seizures 7, 79, 133, 179
self-examination 122

seminal fluid 162
sensation 82
serositis 5, 10
sex 83
sexual drive 90
sexual relations 153–162
sexuality 138, 153
sexually transmitted disease 138
shingles 26
shock 51
sialogues 126
Sjogren's syndrome 153
skin 59–63, 124
skin biopsy 62
skin pigmentation 49
smokers 114
smoking 191
social worker 136, 142, 170
spasticity 145
speech pathologist 142
spermicides 158
spinal cord 72, 75, 141
spinal tap 77, 133
spleen 107, 132
splints 148
sterility 68
steroid myopathy 15
steroids 14, 22, 26, 52, 80, 100, 164,
    165, 177, 182, 190. *See also*
    corticosteroids
stillbirth 163
stress 86
stroke 7, 72, 74, 141, 145, 179, 195
sun exposure 132
sun protection factor 190
sun sensitivity 190
sunburn 59
sunlight 28
sunscreens 10, 59, 134, 190
support 167–172
support group 167, 194
survival 11
syphilis 32, 157

T

T lymphocytes 108
teeth 121–129
telangiectasia 61
temperature method 161
temporomandibular joint (TMJ) 127
Tolectin 134

tolmetin 134
tooth brushing 123, 124, 125
toothbrush 125, 126
toothpaste 124, 125
total hip replacement 119
tranquilizers 89, 154
transfusions 107
treatment 50, 67, 99, 113, 176
trigger 3, 131, 187
Tums 45
twins 40, 188
Tylenol. *See* acetaminophen

U

ulcers 24, 46, 52, 62, 124, 132, 153
ultrasound 146
ultraviolet light 62
urinalysis 133
urine collection, 24 hr 34, 133

V

vagina 62, 95, 157
vaginal dryness 154
vaginal ulcers 153
Valium 89
vasculitis 23, 55, 61, 116, 149
venereal infection 157
vision 49
visual perception 82
vitamin D 65, 114, 190
vitamins 45, 198
vitamins C 97
vitamins E 97
vocational counselor 142
vocational planning services 136, 143

W

walking 148
white blood cells 35, 103, 107

X

Xanax 89
xerostomia 126

Z

Zofran 195

NOTES